The Practice of
Nada Yoga

"With Baird's easy-to-follow instructions, this book offers a practical method to unlock these ancient practices. It is an exciting addition to the vast body of yoga texts."

NANCY GILGOFF, STUDENT OF SRI K. PATTABHI JOIS
AND DIRECTOR OF THE HOUSE OF YOGA & ZEN, MAUI

"Baird, through his many years of practice and study in yoga and in music, has traveled to the depths of nada yoga, the yoga of sound. He leads us, in this remarkable book, to the infinite source of this sacred sound, the Self. If you are a disciplined student of yoga or music, this journey with Baird is an indispensable trip."

BERYL BENDER BIRCH, AUTHOR OF *POWER YOGA*

"Baird's writing voice is strong and sonorous, confidently leading us toward a tranquil mind, an undefended heart, and a more sustained connection with the divine. His meditation exercises are among the clearest and easiest to follow that I have ever read. In a world where sound is associated with stress and overload, *The Practice of Nada Yoga* reminds us, as Baird says, what we might hear if we could listen through God's ears."

GAIL STRAUB, COFOUNDER OF
EMPOWERMENT INSTITUTE AND
AUTHOR OF *RETURNING TO MY MOTHER'S HOUSE*

"Baird Hersey describes in clear, exact steps the process of developing the ancient practice of nada yoga. While these Hindu and Buddhist exercises are often clouded in mystery, he manages to make the process both comprehensible and accessible to Westerners serious about their meditation, contemplation, and concentration practices. This is a book by an experienced practitioner who knows the terrain."

JOSE LUIS STEVENS, PH.D., COFOUNDER OF THE POWER PATH,
AUTHOR OF *AWAKEN THE INNER SHAMAN,* AND COAUTHOR OF
SECRETS OF SHAMANISM AND *THE POWER PATH*

The Practice of
Nada Yoga

Meditation on the
Inner Sacred Sound

Baird Hersey

Inner Traditions
Rochester, Vermont • Toronto, Canada

Inner Traditions
One Park Street
Rochester, Vermont 05767
www.InnerTraditions.com

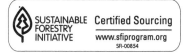

Text stock is SFI certified

Library of Congress Cataloging-in-Publication Data
Hersey, Baird.
  The practice of nada yoga : meditation on the inner sacred sound / Baird Hersey.
     pages cm
  Includes bibliographical references and index.
  ISBN 978-1-62055-181-3 (pbk.) — ISBN 978-1-62055-182-0 (e-book)
  1. Sound—Religious aspects—Hinduism. 2. Meditation—Hinduism. 3. Yoga.
I. Title.
  BL1215.S67H47 2014
  294.5'436—dc23
                                                                    2013020213

Printed and bound in the United States by Lake Book Manufacturing, Inc.
The text stock is SFI certified. The Sustainable Forestry Initiative® program
promotes sustainable forest management.

10 9 8 7 6 5 4 3 2 1

Text design by Virginia Scott Bowman and layout by Priscilla Baker
This book was typeset in Garamond Premier Pro with Gill Sans, Bodoni, and
Galton used as display typefaces
Illustrations by Mavis Gewant. Photographs by Martin Brading.

To send correspondence to the author of this book, mail a first-class letter to the
author c/o Inner Traditions • Bear & Company, One Park Street, Rochester, VT
05767, and we will forward the communication, or contact the author directly at
www.BairdHersey.com.

For Jonji Provenzano
My dear friend and teacher of living and dying
March 27, 1944–September 1, 2008

Throughout this book I make reference to different examples of sound. I have compiled a selection of sound samples to help illustrate some of these examples. Text references with sound accompaniment are indicated with the symbol 𝄢. Please refer to the "Audio List" on page 207 for the Web addresses of these samples.

Contents

PART THREE

Madhyama, the Second Level of Sound

Mind

PART FOUR

Pashyanti, the Third Level of Sound

Visual

PART FIVE

Para, the Fourth Level of Sound

Beyond

PART SIX

The Practice

PART SEVEN

Additive Practices

PART EIGHT

Supportive and Ancillary Practices

PART NINE

A Final Piece

Foreword

By Krishna Das

People ask me, "What is your experience when you chant?" I don't know what to tell them. What I do is a little mystical and mysterious, even to me! I can't even explain it. When I sing I start to release my thoughts and feelings and the stuff of the day. I start to get quieter inside. I am singing to that loving presence that is represented for me by my guru Neem Karoli Baba. I don't necessarily think about him, Maharaj-ji, as a person when I'm singing. It goes deeper than that.

The whole idea of chant is to release ourselves from the obsessive thinking that holds us prisoner. It is not only to be focused on what we are experiencing in that moment. It is to simply chant and allow the practice to work on us. Three hours go by and I can't tell you what happened. I am just the instrument. Maharaj-ji picks up this rusty old pipe and plays beautiful music on it. He puts it down when he's finished, and I go home and watch TV.

Every repetition of the divine names I sing, every single one, is a seed that gets planted. I am scattering seeds. In some sense, Maharaj-ji is using me to plant the seed of the name in everyone who comes. That seed will take root and grow according to its own time, when the situation is ripe. I believe that's Maharaj-ji's way of blessing people and transmitting his love and presence to them. It's completely under the radar and different from what we might experience at the moment. We might feel high or we might feel open or relaxed, but he is transmitting his presence to us through the repetition of the name. My only responsibility is to sing to him and sing to that loving presence with as much intensity and as much sincerity as I can.

Nam, or name, is not necessarily names the way we think of names. These names are roots, root causes of further manifestation. As we repeat these names, or mantras, or make sound with a certain intention, we follow that flow back and in. Through the repetition the flow of thought begins to take the shape of the sound, which is a deeper, more real shape. We gradually become, or realize we are already, in a deeper level, closer to this sound. Nam is the name, the Word, and "in the beginning was the Word." So this sound is what the original name *is*.

When I sang rock and roll, folk music, blues, I was assuming a persona that I felt I needed because I didn't like myself. I was trying very desperately to be someone else. That fulfilled a purpose for me at the time because it allowed me to feel better about myself. I could emulate these blues guys and these rockers and be a person like that. Chanting is about as opposite from that as you can possibly get. The whole purpose of the chanting is to let go of all those personas, to let go of any thoughts about anything, and simply bring your attention back to the sound of the name.

We train ourselves that way, to have that ability to let go of functions throughout the day. We get used to that movement of letting go, that feeling of letting go and coming back to the chant as the object of attention. We acquaint ourselves with the feeling of being released from the obsessive stuff over and over and over and over again. So when the shit does hit the fan and we get a heavy blast of some negative emotion, we have this functioning in us already. That negative emotion may not last a year and a half, it may only last three months. We don't know why we're not feeling as bad as we used to as often as we used to. It is a process that keeps going on. We train ourselves to let go and come back to a deeper and quieter place over and over and over and over and over again.

At the end of an evening of kirtan, there is a deep silence that arises naturally and spontaneously. Saint John of the Cross wrote, "In the

Beginning the Father uttered one Word. That Word is His Son and He utters him forever in everlasting silence. It is in silence that the heart must hear." The silence in the sound is always there. The silence is the absence of the small "self." The silence is the reality.

When people sing and really get into it, they are disappearing. They are enjoying. They're not enjoying that they are enjoying. They are just enjoying. They have left that meta-judgmental thing behind. So when they stop singing, that silence just mushrooms out and blossoms immediately because of the absence of ego-centeredness in the room. That's what sound does.

Sound is a very powerful medium. Our molecules are vibrating and making a sound. The Universe is vibrating and making a sound. Creation is sound. That sound is the movement. It is the beginning of vibration. The first sound is vibration. That is the Om, or *Ah* (the beginning of Om). This cuts right through any kind of psychological bullshit, any kind of version of ourselves that we have. We are essentially a vibration. We are all mixtures of vibration. When we focus on sound itself, it opens up the possibility of dropping down into that deeper level of reality, leaving this one behind.

What Baird Hersey and I do isn't different. When he sings with his group Prana or I sing kirtan, it may look different. But it's very much the same because the intention is the same. I may describe it differently because I'm walking on this path. Baird may describe it differently, but the results are very similar. It's in the fruit that you know what the seed was.

Intention is really the only thing that matters. We are all in these little bubbles of ego. The intention is for the bubble to disappear. When the bubble, the encasing, pops, what happens? The temporary wall between the outside and the inside is gone. Now the outside is the inside and the inside is the outside. The space is one. Oneness is recognized. However it happens, it happens. It's described in different ways by every different being.

We are all moving in the same direction. We are all part of that one being whether we recognize it yet or not. Anything that helps us relax into our true nature is a good path.

Joy is something that Westerners don't have a lot of experience with. We have a lot of experience with pleasure and its opposite, pain. But joy, the simple feeling of well-being, is something that Westerners are really starving for.

This is the essence of the Spiritual Path, the feeling of well-being that already lives in each one of us. It's just so damaged and covered over by our Western psychological shape that it's very hard to do a practice with joy. We are fighting our own tendency to treat ourselves harshly. When we try to do something that is good for ourselves, we recognize that we are our own worst enemy.

It is called *practice* because you've got to do it. You've got to do it when you feel like doing it. You've got to do it when you don't feel like doing it. Because if we only follow our superficial likes and dislikes, we'll never get beyond them. Practice is something we have to do regularly over a period of time in order to relax into a deeper shape, a more real space that lives within us. The best practice is the one that you will do and continue to do because you have to do it.

I was really moved when I read about some of Baird's experiences with the asana practice and with the sound practice. It's exactly what it's supposed to be. It's perfect. He's not doing it because he thinks he should or because it's good for him. He is doing it because it brings him joy.

Baird really goes into the *nada,* the sound. His music led him to that. Most people stop at the music. They don't go into the essence of sound itself. The sound current of the nada definitely dissolves the hard edges and all the personas and all the bullshit. It dissolves it and washes it away. It's like a river of sound, an ocean of sound. It just washes us and cleans us and leaves us unhampered by who we think we are. Or who we thought we were.

What Baird does is clear. It's concise. It's easy to follow. You can

understand the practice and get the results. You don't have to manufac-
ture some idea in your head about it. You do the practice and there is a
result: yoga.

Baird gives a wonderful set of coordinates for people to absorb and
follow. It's the same thing I always say to people: "You don't have to
believe anything first. You don't have to join anything. You don't have
to suspend disbelief. All you have to do is try it. If you like it, you'll do
more." Baird makes the practice clear and accessible to people.

In this book Baird asks, "What would you hear if you could listen
through God's ears?" I think you would hear the everything and the
nothing at the same time. You would hear all the sound and you would
hear the silence in which it is all held. Just like the sky holds everything
within it: the pollution, the beauty, the clouds, the smog, the people, all
the comings and goings. The sky encases everything and holds everything in it. So, all sound is held in the silent sound, the unstruck bell,
the sound of one hand clapping. That silence is alive and full and empty
at the same time. There is nowhere outside of that. There is nowhere to
go. It's here, always here. And so are we.

KRISHNA DAS is one of the foremost devotional singers in the world. He first
traveled to India in 1970, where he met Sri Neem Karoli Baba, through whom
he was introduced to the practice of kirtan devotional chanting.

Introduction

I have always been fascinated by sound. Even as a small child it was a constant source of excitement, joy, and mystery.

One of my earliest memories of live music was my mother taking me to a Memorial Day parade when I was five. Hearing a huge military marching band up close for the first time was absolutely thrilling. When I felt the power of the sound of the massive low brass section, a chill shot up my spine.

At age six I would sit at the piano for hours, playing over and over the three songs my siblings had taught me.

My father used to tell the story of how he came across me one morning listening to a record of "Rudolph the Red-Nosed Reindeer." When he returned five hours later, the song was still playing.

As a child my father studied violin and had planned to become a concert violinist. When he got to college he realized that he also loved writing. He had to choose between spending four hours every day practicing violin or spending that time writing. He chose writing. He made the right choice. He had a long and successful career as a journalist and author. By becoming a musician, in my own way, I have followed his road not taken.

Musical theater composer Richard Rodgers gave me my first "music lesson" when I was six. He sat with me at the piano and had me pick out three notes. I was absolutely awestruck as he took the three notes I had tentatively chosen and instantly made them into a song. He then told my father he thought I had musical talent. We all knew where the talent truly lay.

My formal musical training began when I was seven. I took lessons on a small wooden flute called a recorder. I was a terrible student. Because I never practiced, my lessons were little more than me noodling around trying to find the right notes. When I was nine I sang and played recorder in music classes at school. By this time I had overcome my own propensity for noodling and had a very low tolerance for the noodlings of others. I guess we most dislike in others the failings that we carry in ourselves.

It was the days of the Hi-Fi and my father put together a good one for playing LPs. The house was always filled with music: Rachmaninov, Mozart, Bach, Miles Davis, Dave Brubeck, The Modern Jazz Quartet, Odetta, The Weavers, Josh White, "Oklahoma," "My Fair Lady," "The Music Man," and many, many others.

My family also owned a small reel-to-reel tape recorder that I commandeered for my own use. As well as recording music I did sound experiments, such as recording dripping water and playing it back at a higher speed to bring out its rhythmic patterns. My mother would recount how, as a child, I had played melodies on the standing radiator in my room by hitting different parts of it with sticks. She took me to many wonderful concerts and shows, among them Ravi Shankar, Ray Charles, Howlin' Wolf, Leonard Bernstein's Young People's Concerts, Marcel Marceau, and many Broadway shows. At the original production of the "Music Man," I was shushed by a man sitting in front of me for singing along with all of the songs I had heard so many times on our Hi-Fi at home.

The music of the late 1950s and early 1960s played continuously on my green Zenith "Racetrack" radio that was a hand-me-down from my older brother. The music of Brenda Lee, Jackie Wilson, The Flamingos, Sam Cooke, Patti Page, and The Everly Brothers, all drew my ear and provided a refuge for me. I wrapped their sound around me like a comfortable, warm blanket to give solace to my preadolescent heart.

I started playing my first real instrument, clarinet, when I was thirteen. I then moved on to saxophone. The following year I took up guitar to fill a vacancy in a rock band at my high school.

As a teenager I was fortunate to witness the beginning of one of the most important cultural phenomena of the twentieth century: The Beatles. I was at their first public performance in the United States. It is widely believed that the first time they played in America was the Sunday night broadcast of *The Ed Sullivan Show*. In fact, it took place at a rehearsal on that same day and was much longer and more involved than the show that aired that evening.

Seeing them play, hearing their sound come to life, watching the reaction around me, all made me wonder, *what is it about sound that is so powerful?*

In 1968 I worked on the film crew for *Monterey Pop*, a documentary about the very first rock festival that took place in Monterey, California. When I wasn't recording sound with one of the camera crews, I watched the performances of Otis Redding, Ravi Shankar, Jimi Hendrix, The Who, Booker T and the MGs, The Grateful Dead, Jefferson Airplane, Paul Butterfield Blues Band, and many others. Again, I wondered what it was about making sound that was so impactful to the thousands of people gathered for the festival.

From that point forward I dedicated myself to becoming a musician. In my senior year in high school, and then in college, I studied composing, orchestration, arranging, and guitar. I then went on to a career in music, writing and playing in many different styles. I have played in rock bands, led a jazz big band, composed symphonic and choral music, written music for TV, and I now lead a nine-voice vocal group, Prana. In a career that has spanned more than fifty years, I have recorded twelve albums.

When I was twenty-two there was a moment while I was playing guitar that both fascinated and confounded me. I was playing in a jam session with some friends when all of a sudden I felt like "I" wasn't there anymore. I had connected so completely with the sound, it was as if I had become part of it. This was not a chemically induced experience. Somehow I had gotten out of the way and the sound was flowing through me. I tried to recapture that moment time and time again without success. I knew that this was one of the answers to the questions I had been asking about the power of sound and its effect on people. It wasn't until many years later when I started practicing yoga asana that I again discovered how to become the instrument through which the music is played.

When I was in my early twenties without any kind of formal training, I would sit cross-legged, close my eyes, and just listen to the sound of the ocean. I would try to become one with it although I had no idea what that really meant or how to accomplish it. A friend mentioned she had seen me sitting on a rock by the water meditating. I thought to myself, "Meditating? I'm not meditating. I'm just listening."

In college I became interested in Tibetan monastic music. There was something about it that I found highly compelling. It was both uplifting and mystifying. It had a power that I hadn't experienced before: the power to transform. One day while I was listening through headphones to a recording of the low gravelly voices of Tibetan monks chanting, I kept hearing fire engine sirens in my neighborhood. When I took off the headphones, I realized it wasn't fire engines at all. It was the monks. They were making high whistling tones three and four octaves above their low vocal sound.

After college when I was recruiting players for my big band, I invited a talented saxophonist named Yoshi Maruta to my house. I played recordings of some of my music and music from around the world that had influenced me. After listening he said to me, "Music for you is religion." I was surprised by his comment. He was reflecting back to me what was obvious to him but not to me. In my approach to music, what I composed and performed had begun to embody a respect for the spiritual nature of sound. There is no doubt that the spiritual aspect of music eventually led me to asana practice.

For me, yoga and music have always been intertwined. My first yoga practice was in 1988. I wrote some music for a meditation tape for a yoga teacher named Marcia Albert. In return she gave me some asana classes. From the very beginning it was clear to me that asana practice had a powerful transformational quality similar to what I was looking for in music.

At the end of the very first class I took with Marcia, as I lay in *shavasana* (corpse pose), I fell into a deep relaxation and lost consciousness. After a few minutes I woke up. Not wanting to seem impatient I continued to lie still with my eyes closed, looking straight ahead. I began to see brilliant clouds of colored light. Green, aqua blue, and indigo light, each in turn danced before my closed eyes. For many years after that I would ask yoga teachers what had caused this. What had been opened in my body to make this happen? No one knew.

Right around this time two good friends helped me move forward into overtone singing. First, percussionist and vocalist David Moss, knowing I was interested in Tibetan music, gave me some insight into how the monks make those high whistling tones. He said, "You know Baird, if you just put the tip of your tongue in the roof of your mouth like this, you can make overtones."

Second, Tom Guralnick, a saxophonist and New Music promoter, sent me a recording of Tuvan throat singing that also uses overtones. The presence and strength of the overtone was not only an inspiration but was highly instructive.

With these two pieces of new information I began to teach myself the basic technique of overtone singing, vocally producing two pitches at once. While singing one note with the vocal chords, you use your tongue, lips, and jaw to tune the vibrating air in your throat and mouth to produce a second higher pitch. As I began singing overtones I was constantly drawn back to the purity of their sound. As I practiced more and more, I began to hear the faintest glimmer of the transformational quality I had heard in the chanting of the Tibetan monks.

At the same time I was trying out various different lineages of yoga asana. In 1997 I was introduced to ashtanga yoga. During my first practice of ashtanga I thought, "This is what I've been looking for." It felt like I had come home. Again, at the end of that first practice I had another unique experience.

As I sat in *bandha padhmasana* (bound lotus), a jolt of what felt like electric current shot from the base of my spine up to the top of my head filling my body with an intense blissful feeling. I was mystified by what had happened. I was afraid that if I talked about it people would think I was either crazy, or worse, being boastful.

As asana was beginning to transform me, I started working even more seriously on overtone singing to bring out the deeper transformational quality in the sound. Overtones are perfectly aligned frequencies that do not exist in Western music tuning. The perfection of the relationship of these pitches affects us on a physical, mental, and spiritual level. The perfect symmetry of these vibrations relaxes the body, stills the mind, and opens the heart. Their sound holds the power to transform that I had been looking for.

After about a year of ashtanga classes and workshops, I started a daily home practice. During that period I did music for yoga workshops and meditation tapes. In the days and weeks after doing an ashtanga Intermediate Series workshop, I felt as though the practice had cracked open the shell around my heart. I was filled with an overwhelming feeling of joyful love. This revelation turned my life upside down.

Within a month of that Intermediate Series workshop, I recorded *Waking the Cobra,* an overtone singing chakra meditation CD. I originally recorded it as a Christmas gift for twelve friends. Most of these friends were yoga teachers. Many of them started playing the CD in their classes. Their students began asking me for copies. Initially I was just burning individual discs on my computer, but the recording took on a life of its own. The demand became so great that I had to have a large run of copies printed.

Over the next couple of years I let go of much of my previous life. Among the many things that changed was the kind of music I was composing. Making meditation music was not something that I chose to do. It chose me. Letting go of guitar, an instrument I had played for more than thirty-five years, was not something I'd planned to do. It wasn't that I decided to lay the guitar down, I just never picked it up.

My main musical focus became overtone singing. It gave me such an immediate connection with the sound. As I sang I became part of the sound. It flowed through me. As I sang I continuously felt that same connection that in all my years of playing the guitar, I had only experienced once.

In 2000 I met and studied with Pattabhi Jois, the guru of ashtanga yoga. I knew immediately that I had found my teacher. I studied with him for nine years, both in Mysore, India, and here in the United States. His teaching continued to open my body and my mind.

As my life continued to unfold, experiences that had lain dormant and unresolved began to resurface. The transformational quality of sound, the bright colored clouds of internal light, the bliss of energy shooting up my spine, the opening of my heart, these were all experiences that began to coalesce and draw my attention. For many years all four of these experiences had raised a multitude of unanswered questions. These experiences were now beginning to align as signposts on a path straight toward the practice of nada yoga.

Ever since I started doing yoga asana and singing overtones, I had been interested in learning nada yoga. I had been working on finding the transformational quality of external sound through overtone singing, but I also wanted to explore the divine quality of internal sound. I went to many workshops and studied with many teachers. Much of what I was taught as nada yoga was based on the *ragas,* improvisation on the scales and patterns of North Indian classical music. Although this is a rich and fruitful field of study, it wasn't what I was looking for. I was seeking the path to the internal sound.

When I would ask, "What is the *nada?*" I was often told, "God is in the note." This answer was followed by the playing of a note with a great amount of feeling. This, of course, is true. It is what I was beginning to discover through overtone singing, but it was not the only answer I was looking for. I was also looking for the key to *anahata nada,* the unstruck sound, the eternal sound that is in all of us and connects us with the greater Universe.

I read a great deal. Even though I was reading about some of the very practices I do today, at that time they seemed simplistic. It seemed to me there had to be more to it than just listening.

It is said that we can only hear a teaching when we are ready to hear it. For many years I just wasn't ready to hear the teaching, not until I started to look more thoroughly at the *Hatha Yoga Pradipika*. At that moment all of my practices, my hunger to learn, and the information contained in the instruction all came together.

While preparing to take a teaching on the *Hatha Yoga Pradipika*, I studied the text in more depth than I ever had before. I realized that in my reading I had never gotten to the fourth chapter. Halfway through the chapter I came upon the phrase, "Here now begins the teaching of nada yoga." I was a little shocked and pleasantly surprised. As I read on I had the feeling of finally discovering the key to the world of internal sound I had been seeking.

I started doing the practices described in the text. At every step I was awed by the depth that was available through these practices. What I discovered while sitting in meditation would send me back to the text for clarification. This in turn led me to even deeper levels of discovery. This drove me to look further into other ancient texts containing teachings on nada yoga. Some of the very texts I had dismissed as simplistic provided corroboration and expansion of the instructions I had found in the *Hatha Yoga Pradipika*.

Countless times I would have a direct experience in a meditation and then, within a day or two, find a verse in one of the texts that would not only confirm my experience but instruct me as to what to do next.

The sounds of the nada as described in the *Hatha Yoga Pradipika* were so familiar to me. They were an internal reflection of the external sound I had been spending so many years studying and practicing: overtone singing. The whistling, whirring, thundering sounds of ocean surf, waterfall, bell, conch shell, horn, flute, tinkling chimes, bees, and crickets were almost identical to the sound of the overtones that I had been cultivating in the music I was composing and performing.

As I delved into the text and practiced, I again had the feeling of arriving home. I had finally found the meditation practice I had been seeking for so many years. I had finally found the answers to my questions. What were the brilliant clouds of colored light I had seen? What was the electric current that shot from the base of my spine up to the top of my head filling me with bliss? What caused my heart to open as I practiced ashtanga yoga? Most importantly, what was the source of the transformational power of sound? I may not have found the answer to Life, but I'd certainly found some of the answers for my life. They were all there in the text and the practice that it taught.

Through the practice of this meditation I have reached levels of introspection I never thought possible for me. I have experienced a quiet mind, an uplifted spirit, and bliss. What does this bliss feel like? It is a tingling, energetic, pleasantly electric feeling in body and mind. It is a feeling of simultaneous joyful expectation and wondrous release. Like yoga asana practice, bliss is not an end in itself. Once attained, we mustn't get too attached to it. It is not enlightenment. It is, however, a step in that direction. It is a place to begin.

Although instruction on nada meditation is readily available, it is not a practice that is widely taught. It is in some ways a lost practice.

The second half of the fourth chapter of the *Hatha Yoga Pradipika* is instruction on nada yoga. It is based on the teachings of Gorakshanath (or Gorakhnath), a yogi who lived in the late eleventh and early twelfth centuries. He traveled and gathered yogic practices, which he codified into numerous texts. The *Hatha Yoga Pradipika,* later compiled by Swami Svatmarama, includes Gorakshanath's teaching on nada yoga.

The heart of my book is based on the *Hatha Yoga Pradipika* and many other texts (excerpts of which are listed at the end of the book*). When brought together these texts gather four meditations into one.

---

*In this book I have included source texts that are relevant to the practice of nada yoga. I have presented these texts in language that is accessible and easily understood as instruction, rather than their literal translations. In some cases I have included only what is pertinent to the daily practice. (See Appendix: The Source Texts.)

They are meditations on finding bliss through stillness, opening our heart to unconditional love, seeing the Internal Divine Light, and hearing the Inner Sacred Sound. They are the four components of this form of nada yoga. Each one, individually, is a powerful meditation. When done together the positive result is exponential. Each of the four aspects supports and deepens the others.

All the meditations and practices in this book come from my direct experiences. I have drawn on my life as a musician and composer to share what I know about sound. Parts one through four provide meditations on learning to listen to sound in new ways. They are preparation for parts five and six, which focus on the daily meditation practice of nada yoga based on the *Hatha Yoga Pradipika* and other texts. Part seven inserts some additional pieces into the daily practice. These additions will deepen and expand its effect. Part eight provides supportive and ancillary practices that are done independent of the daily meditation. Each is a practice of its own. They will help broaden, strengthen, and support the practice of nada yoga.

I am no master. I only teach what I know. I teach what others have taught me and what I have learned through my own experiences. Of course, practice is the foundation. Experimentation, failure, vulnerability, and contemplation are all also very important. Most important of all is an unending curiosity about the Divine that exists within all human beings and the possibility to open our hearts and share unconditional love.

Something has shifted for me since I started doing this meditation. I feel as though I have been given a beautiful gift. That is why I have written this book, to share this gift of comfort, peace, and the blissful connection between the Universe within us and the Universe that surrounds us.

I have emphasized again and again in this book that this is an experiential practice, not an intellectual one. It is not some esoteric exercise with an unattainable result. It is not a practice only to be analyzed, conceptualized, contextualized, or theorized about. Quite simply, it is a practice to be done.

As with asana, it is both a practice of self-discovery and the discovery of an ancient path tread by sages and yogis many centuries ago. We make these discoveries by experiencing them, not reading about them. So, don't go by what I say. Do the practice. Try it for yourself. See if you get results. See if it works for you. If it does, then go deeper.

PART ONE

Overview

1 ✸ Listen!

Here now begins the teaching of nada yoga as taught by Gorakshanath, accessible to all, even those with no experience of yoga.

HATHA YOGA PRADIPIKA 4.65

When you finish reading this sentence sit quietly for a few minutes with your eyes closed and just listen.

You have just finished your first practice of nada yoga!

What did you hear?
How long did you listen?
What distracted you?
Were you able to go back to listening?

2 ✳ What Is Nada Yoga?

One who desires true union of yoga should leave all thinking behind and concentrate with single-pointed attention on the nada.

HATHA YOGA PRADIPIKA 4.93

You have lost your way. You were walking down a country road. It started to get foggy. It started to get dark. Now you find yourself walking across open country unable to see more than a few feet in front of you. What is the right direction? How will you find your way home?

As it gets darker you worry that you are straying farther and farther from your destination. The fear begins to well up inside of you, "I'm lost and will never get home." Then you remember your home and those who love you waiting there for you. You feel love in your heart. You let it grow. You find you are no longer fearful.

You hear a sound in the distance. It is not recognizable, but it is familiar. You move toward it, but it is muted as it echoes through the fog. It is difficult to tell exactly where it's coming from. Uncertain, you continue forward.

Dimly at first, out of the darkness, you begin to see a faint flickering light. As you move toward it, it begins to glow more brightly. It becomes a fixed point of radiant light.

As you get closer you recognize the sound as the voice of someone who loves and cares about you. They are calling your name. As you move toward them, you realize you can see, through the windows of

17

your living room, the light of a fire burning warm and bright in the fireplace. You have found your way home to the love of your family and the comfort of a cozy fire.

Every day we try to find our way through the fog of distractions in the world around us. We search for any sound to show us the way, any light that indicates what direction we should take.

In nada yoga the calling voice is the Inner Sacred Sound.[1] The warm, bright fire is the Internal Divine Light. Together they show us the way home and our connection to all things everywhere.

Nada yoga is the yoga of listening. It is a way to turn inward on a journey that may eventually lead you to enlightenment, but at the very least, nada yoga will fill your daily life with comfort, contentment, and what some call bliss. In nada yoga sound is more than what is heard through our ears. It is an internal sound that is not perceived by our external sense organs. By focusing our mind on this internal sound we re-unite our essential self with the eternal and the infinite. In this re-union we find bliss in both the body and the mind.

Nada yoga is ancient. It dates back to the *Rig-Veda,* which is three-and-a-half centuries old. The *Rig-Veda* is a set of Indian verses in Sanskrit. It is one of the world's oldest religious texts. In it we find the *Nada-Bindu Upanishad.* It teaches meditation on the nada, the Inner Sacred Sound. Much of that text was later incorporated into the *Hatha Yoga Pradipika.*

NADA

Nad is a Sanskrit word, which means to sound, thunder, roar, howl, or cry. Adding an "*a*" at its end makes it *nada,* which means sound or tone. *Nada* also means river or stream. If we put these different meanings together, "stream" and "to sound," we have the object of meditation in nada yoga, an internal "sound stream."

Scientists now tell us the entire Universe and everything in it is vibrating. That vibration is the core of what connects and coheres everything. Vibration is sound. Many ancient texts hold this same view. Everything is vibrating. Everything is sound. As Hazrat Inayat Khan says in *The Mysticism of Sound and Music*: "[T]hat which has created, and which is holding, and in which is held the whole manifestation and the whole cosmos, is one power, and that is vibration."[2]

This Universal Vibration is without beginning or end, reaching infinitely from before the Big Bang into the unending future. Even today as the planets move through space, they are vibrating. The sun in the sky is vibrating at millions of different frequencies. The gravitational waves emanating from black holes, expanding and contracting space, are vibrations. Vibration is everywhere and permeates and connects everything. This is Universal Consciousness. Vast, pervasive, interconnected, constant, it is that which enlivens everything. Reverend Jaganath Carrera puts it this way in *Inside the Yoga Sutras*: "Nada . . . The first vibration out of which all creation manifests. Sound is the first manifestation of the Absolute Brahman. . . ."[3]

In the same way, each of us is vibrating on many levels. We are vibrating from the subatomic to the cellular level, from the rhythm of our respiration to the pulse of our heart, from the vibrational tension of our muscles to the microelectrical pulses of our nervous system.

There is also within us a vibration, an internal sound. This is the nada. Khan said: "[E]ach person has his note . . . that particular note is expressive of his life's evolution, expressive of his soul, of the condition of his feelings and of his thoughts."[4]

For each person this sound may be different, yet it is all part of the vibration of the Universe. We are all part of the Sacred Sound Stream. The nada is constant, ever present. It is always there, both within us and reaching into the greater Universe. All we have to do is listen.

We seek this stream of sound, patiently waiting for it with joyful anticipation. Once it has arisen in our awareness, it is where we place our attention. This is the practice of nada yoga. We follow the river of sound, which carries us to an ocean of bliss.

BINDU

The meaning of *bindu* is both physical and metaphysical. The literal translation is "point," "drop," or "dot." It is generally understood to mean "seed" point or point of concentration of power.

The most widely known bindu is the dot over the Om symbol. It indicates the silent echo out of which the sound of Om will arise again.

A yantra is a geometric visual symbol used in tantric meditation and astrology. In most yantras there is a bindu. It is the center point. It is the place from which the yantra begins. A circle is drawn with a string or a tool with the bindu at its center. It is also the center point of meditation on the yantra, an entryway into Universal Consciousness.

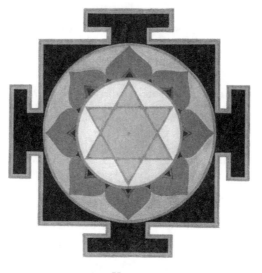

Yantra

Bindu is also the potential for creation. It is the point at which the capacity for the unmanifest to become manifest is realized. It is a nucleus or "egg" where prana and consciousness, Shakti and Shiva, space and time, seed and ovum come together: the rejoining of these halves into a whole causing the surge of creation.

There are many opinions as to exactly where in the human body the bindu physically resides. Hindu priests, though their heads are shaved, have one small patch of hair at the top of the back of their heads. In paintings of ancient yogis, their hair is often in a topknot. Both of these are outward physical expressions of the internal bindu.

Many spiritual texts site the bindu between the eyebrows or behind the center of the forehead. Others place it deep in the heart. Some texts also equate it with the uvula, the "bell" that hangs from the soft palate at the back of the mouth. Some believe it is the pineal gland, which is in the center of the brain at the top of the brain stem.

Tibetan Buddhists believe there are three drops: one at the crown of the head, one at the heart, and one at the navel.

At the time of the collation of the *Hatha Yoga Pradipika,* bindu also meant "light" or "radiant point." The *Goraksha Paddhati* refers to that light as the *Nila Bindu,* "the blue dot." It states that "Focusing between the brows will manifest the Nila Bindu." Swami Muktananda, guru of siddha yoga, called this the "Blue Pearl," and talked about its qualities: "The blue light is the light of all lights. . . . The blue light is the light that illuminates the mind, that illuminates everything."⁵

As we progress into nada yoga, we find that the bindu as light becomes as important as the sound itself. The bindu is a portal through which we find the nada and reconnect our individual consciousness with Universal Consciousness.

YOGA

Here in the West, when we think of yoga, we usually think of hatha yoga, the practice of a series of physical postures. There are other forms of yoga that are not physical practices.

- Karma yoga, the yoga of action through helping others.
- Bhakti yoga, the yoga of devotion through ritual and chant.
- Jnana yoga, the yoga of knowledge through education and thought.
- Raja yoga, the yoga of meditation by turning the mind inward.

To "yoke," "join," "attach," "harness" are literal translations of the Sanskrit word *yoga*. In its philosophical sense, yoga means to join in union, to "become one with." It is the realization of non-dualism, where the illusion of separation between "I" and the rest of the Universe is removed so we recognize them as one. This concept can be distilled down to its essence in the Vedantic phrase *Tat tvam asi,* "You are that." This means your consciousness and the Universal Consciousness are one and the same: no difference, no division.

With the practice of nada yoga, we take away the illusion that we are all separate. By following the radiance of the Divine Light and the vibration of the Sacred Sound, we strive to enter into union (yoga) and realize the blissful reconnection of our consciousness with the all-encompassing Universal Consciousness.

3 ✳ Practice Makes Perfect

Through listening to the nada for fifteen days the yogi overcomes all obstacles and feels blissful.

HATHA YOGA PRADIPIKA 4.83

WHY PRACTICE NADA YOGA?

The practice of nada yoga is not complex or complicated. It is amazingly simple. It is the act of listening, initially externally and eventually internally.

What keeps us from listening? The distractions offered up by our mind with blinding speed and deafening variety, our mind chatter. Our monkey mind jumps from thought to thought: *What will I have for breakfast? . . . That was a nice meal I had with . . . I wonder if they got that job . . . Am I going to lose my job? . . . Do I have my wallet? . . . It sure cost a lot to fix my car . . . Ohh, my foot fell asleep . . . It would be nice to take a nap . . .* and on and on.

We often spend so much time in our heads worrying, hoping, remembering, and planning that sometimes we miss out on life going on around us. As Mark Twain said, "Some of the worst things in my life never happened!"

So, the initial step is learning to listen without interrupting ourselves. This is the single most important premise of this practice: if we are actively *listening*, we can't be talking, even inside our heads. As we move through the four levels of sound, we will learn how to focus our mind on listening so that we alleviate distraction.

Having cleared away the mind chatter, we then can find union with the nada. A quiet mind is a peaceful mind. A peaceful mind is a place where joy and bliss naturally arise.

The practice of nada yoga is quickly and easily learned. Its rewarding, uplifting benefits are experienced from the very beginning. Once the basics are mastered, we can carry them with us throughout our day and use them to bring us into the present moment; we can use them to live the life we want to live.

With regular daily practice, in a relatively short time, we can experience deep levels of meditation that will bring comfort, calm, and contentment to our daily life. We experience being part of something larger than ourselves. We come to understand that we are one and the same with the Universe. We are not only connected to, but are one with, all things everywhere.

Nada yoga is not an intellectual pursuit. It is an experiential practice. The discoveries we make are through doing the practice, rather than thinking about it. As my teacher Sri K. Pattabhi Jois used to say: "Practice! Practice! Practice!" "Ninety-nine percent practice, one percent theory." "Do your practice and all is coming." Although he was teaching ashtanga yoga, the very same principle applies to nada yoga as well.

4 ✳ The Four Levels of Sound

Put the self in the sound and the sound in the self. When the self is sound all else falls away.

GHERANDA SAMHITA 7.8

The structure of the four levels of sound came from philosophers and linguists of the Vedic period in ancient India. It was handed down through the Vedas and the *Kundalini Upanishads*. It is an attempt to understand and codify the process of speech.

When a person is about to speak they begin with the highest and most subtle level, *para* ("beyond") sound. It is pure intention without word or form. This then leads to the next lower level, *pashyanti* ("visual") sound. At the pashyanti level the person is forming intention into an idea. When they internally make that thought into words, it is at the third level, *madhyama* ("between" thought and sound). The final or grossest level, *vaikhari* ("utterance"), is the word or sound spoken into the external world to express the thought.

If we think of the four levels as a stairway, the process of the formation of speech descends those stairs. Moving from the most subtle level, para, down through less and less subtle levels, pashyanti, then madhyama, to end at the gross level, vaikhari.

To apply these four levels more broadly to sound, we will, instead, ascend the same stairway. We move up from the gross level, vaikhari, to the most subtle, para.

25

THE FOUR LEVELS OF SOUND

Speech				Sound
Para				Para
	Pashyanti		Pashyanti	
		Madhyama	Madhyama		
		Vaikhari	Vaikhari		

This progression takes us from the outer world of sound to the inner world of the nada. When we arrive at the highest level we connect our individual internal sound with the omnipresent sound of the Universe.

VAIKHARI

The 1st Level of Sound

This first level is the sound in the external world around us, any sound that we can perceive through our ears.

This includes the thousands of sounds that we hear every day, regardless of whether we focus on them or filter them out. We hear and pay attention to language, music, our alarm clock, cell phone, computer, appliances, and many other sound cues in our daily life.

There are also the sounds in our ambient environment. Some are active and easy to hear. More subtle are the passive sounds. These are acoustics and resonant frequencies, which give a sound made in our living room a very different quality than when it is made in our shower. More subtle still are the many internal sounds that our bodies physically make. We filter them out in order to hear the other sounds in our surroundings that we want to focus on.

MADHYAMA

The 2nd Level of Sound

The second level of sound encompasses the sounds of the mind, any sound that we can imagine or recall and hear in our mind.

Our brain has stored in it thousands and thousands of sounds. We know or recognize many songs and countless specific sounds. Some of these may have an emotional or intellectual meaning for us.

We may remember a poem we recited in third grade or the words someone said to us at an important moment in our lives. A song that was meaningful to us at a specific time may bring back other memories from that same period. Some of us have an inner voice or dialogue that may encourage us, warn us, or criticize us. We may sometimes get stuck in a repetition of self-admonishment or a tape loop of a conversation we once had.

As mentioned, *madhyama* means "between." Sound memories are a bridge between the outside world and our inner world. The same neural pathways within our brains are activated when we recall a sound as were activated when we originally heard that sound. The difference is that instead of using our ears, the sound is reassembled from our memory.

PASHYANTI
The 3rd Level of Sound

When reading a novel words can paint a vivid picture. On the radio sound effects are used to help us visualize a place or circumstance. On television sound effects are used in the same way to enhance an on-screen location or represent off-camera action.

The pashyanti, or the visual level of sound, is where the visual world and auditory world intersect, overlap, and eventually merge.

First, it is sound pictures: visuals of an object, place, or person summoned by a specific sound. Even a place or situation we may not have experienced can be built by sound. Sounds can provide a pathway through our memory that triggers parts of a picture we then assemble into a whole.

Second, it is possible to hear an abstract sound, such as instrumental music, and generate a visual narrative like an internal movie. We do this with our intuitive imagination. We get a feeling from the music and imagine a scene to go with it.

Going a step further, we can construct an abstract picture of the sound itself. It is a picture that is not identifiable as an object in the real world. It can be either a visual of the whole sound or visual representations of the notes played by the individual instruments, all finding their own place in the totality of the visual/auditory landscape.

This intersection, overlap, or merger can flow both ways. Not only can a sound generate a visual, but a visual can generate a sound. An internal picture of someone we remember may cross over into hearing something they said. Any visual, moving, or still image can have its own soundtrack in our mind.

PARA
The 4th Level of Sound

Para, "beyond," can be understood in a number of ways in this context: beyond words, beyond sound, the voice beyond, going beyond our sense organs, beyond what we have reached before, beyond what we know, beyond our imagination, beyond ourselves.

Para is the inner perception of our connection to something greater than ourselves. We move beyond the external world of sounds around us. We move beyond our sound memories, beyond our internal dialogue, beyond our sound imaginings, to an inner listening for a sound that is always present within us: an Inner Sacred Sound Stream that, should we choose to ride it, will carry us to bliss and then even further into higher realms of consciousness.

THE FOUR LEVELS OF SOUND

Level	Translation	Speech	Sound
Para	Beyond	Intention	Transcendent
Pashyanti	Visual	Abstract thoughts	Color/form
Madhyama	Between	Concrete thoughts	Mental
Vaikhari	Utterance	Verbalized	External

5 ✳ Before We Begin

Practice is the foundation of stillness when sustained with devotion through time.

YOGA SUTRAS 1.14

Here are a few ideas that might be helpful in your approach to meditation:

1. **Set a time.** Choose a time every day when you can have some uninterrupted time to yourself without the usual distractions. Setting a length of time to meditate may allow you not to rush.
2. **Choose a place.** Find a place in your home to meditate that isn't used for anything else. Set up an altar with a picture or two of teachers or someone who has had a positive effect on your life. Make it a sacred space. When you go there, you will automatically transition into a meditative mode. Don't meditate in your bedroom. It is good to put some physical distance between your sitting and your sleeping.
3. **Find symmetry.** Sit comfortably with your back straight and the right side of your body in the same position as the left side.
4. **Close your eyes.** In order to limit external visual distractions, close your eyes after reading the instruction for each meditation.
5. **Start with the breath.** Focus on your breath, becoming aware of both the inhale and exhale.
6. **Let go of distractions.** If they do come up, either from your surroundings or from within your mind, notice them but don't engage

in them. Bring yourself back to your point of attention. Notice these distractions as you would notice clouds passing in an open sky.

7. **Be compassionate with yourself.** Treat yourself as you would treat someone else who has had no experience with what you are teaching them. Rather than judging yourself (*I can't do this . . . I'm awful at this . . . I'm never going to be able to do this . . .*), notice the small incremental refinements that happen over time.

8. **See, feel, smell, taste, hear your way in.** We all perceive, process, and learn from the world around us in our own way. Some of us look at the world and make pictures. Some of us touch the world and get feelings. Some of us listen to the world and hear sounds. Some of us combine two or more of the senses. If you have difficulty with any of the meditations, start with whatever sense you are most comfortable with. From there cross over into the world of sound.

9. **Be playful. Experiment.** Try new things you didn't think you could do. Don't be afraid to fail. Failure is one of the ways we learn. The most important note in composing a melody is often when your finger slips and the "wrong" note you play opens up a whole new world of possibilities.

10. **Find the joy.** By practicing you are taking care of yourself. That is an important and joyful thing. Finding that joy will help you return to your practice time and time again.

11. **Leave your *self* out of it.** Turn the process and outcome over to a higher power, the connection between all things, or the Universe. Become only the flute through which the song pours.

12. **Run, Baby, Run!** If you were going to run a marathon, you wouldn't go out and run twenty miles the first day of training. In the same way, training your mind to have endurance in meditation takes time. Be patient. Over time your ability to stay focused will come.

13. **Make it a habit.** To progress in any practice it is important to make it a regular, sustained daily event. If you do, bliss will quickly be attained.

PART TWO

Vaikhari, the First Level of Sound

External

6 ✺ How We Hear

He who knows the secret of the sounds, knows the mystery
of the whole universe.

HAZRAT INAYAT KHAN

High in the hills, green with grass, a lone Tuvan herder looks after his flock of sheep. He hears the low moan and high whistle of the wind wrapping itself around the rocks in an overhanging cliff above him. He begins to sing and his voice, incredibly, is making two sounds at once: one, a low continuous drone and above it, a high fluty whistle. He pauses after a breath's worth of singing and listens to the wind in the rocks above him. Then, as if in conversation, he begins to sing again.

As the sun rises high in the sky he hears a cricket close by in the grass. He sings again, this time with a lower drone; the high whistle is a scratchy sustain. His singing is punctuated by the listening that every good conversation demands.

As the long light and stillness of sunset spreads across the valley, he hears the rumble and rush of the river far below him in the valley. He answers with a low drone with a repeated quick rhythmic arc above it.

In addition to the sound of the rocks, wind, cricket, and river, he also has songs for the summer breeze, the falling rain, the chirping of a bird, the thud of a horse's hooves, and the gurgle of a stream. His listening focuses on each specific sound. He filters out all other surrounding sounds. He imitates, echoes, and merges with the sounds in his natural sonic environment. *9* (See page 207.)

HOW WE HEAR

1. A vibration or sound happens in our surroundings. The vibration causes pressure waves. They travel through the air and enter the ear canal.

2. The waves cause the eardrum to vibrate. This causes small bones within the ear to move. This in turn causes the fluid in the inner ear to vibrate. Within that fluid are micro-hairs. If the vibration is a frequency that stimulates a hair sensitive to that frequency, it produces a neurotransmitter that travels to the brain in the form of an electrical impulse.

3. The brain sorts the impulse, comparing and contrasting it to previous impulses in order to recognize or categorize it.

4. The brain then reacts according to the sound's relationship to previous sounds and their effect or meaning. Some sounds are filtered out, some focused on.

5. The intellect makes a judgment about those it is focused on. It prioritizes how they should be interpreted, attended to, or acted upon.

6. The specifics of the sound are then stored to be recalled or used as reference for comparison for future incoming sound.

7 ❋ Filtering

Music is the silence between the notes.

CLAUDE DEBUSSY

There are literally thousands and thousands of bits of information flying into our brain every second. From all the reflections of light and color entering our eyes, to the millions of nerve cells in our body sending information about temperature, texture, pressure, balance, and vibration to the myriad of smells that enter our nose with every breath, to the panorama of audible sounds that surround us, we are inundated with stimuli. If we paid attention to it all we would be overwhelmed, immobilized, and unable to function. So, our brain has instantaneous and precise routines for prioritizing information so that we immediately know what we should focus our attention on and what we should filter out and disregard.

Out of the corner of our eye, we see something slither through the grass near our foot. We hear a loud noise. We smell smoke or feel something crawling up our back under our shirt. Because survival is at the top of the list of unconscious priorities, our attention immediately shifts to whatever may be threatening us. Simultaneously, we filter out all other input.

I lived in the city for ten years. After working intensely on an album project, recording, listening, and mixing every day for weeks, I took a vacation in the country. There was no television, radio, or anything to play recorded music on. This was well before the day of cell phones and laptop computers. The quiet of the country overwhelmed me. I couldn't sleep with all that quiet.

I was used to the daily bombardment of the sounds of the city: some of it purposeful and some made just by neglect. I was used to filtering it all out. I had learned to sublimate the sonic overload. Now that I wasn't experiencing this stimulation, my brain didn't know what to do.

In the rainforest, when a predator is near, all the birds and animals fall silent. Some primal part of my brain was responding to the silence. My survival mode was saying, if there is no sound, something must be wrong. My filters, which allowed me to sleep in the city, had nothing to filter out. They were waking me up because *no noise* signaled danger. After a week my filters had adjusted and I began to sleep more normally.

Since that time I have lived in the quiet of the country for twenty-five years. On a recent visit to the city I stayed in a room facing a busy street. At first I was not able to sleep because of the noise on the street. Every time a truck rumbled by or a motorcycle engine revved as it raced up the street or a bus caused the building to shudder and rattle, I woke up. Again, after a couple of days I began to acclimate. The filters began to come up and I didn't wake up so much.

This first exercise is meant to wake up our external listening, to help us let go of some of our filters. It will help us to hear all the sounds of the world around us with more subtlety.

✸ Ambient Sound Meditation

It may be helpful to close your eyes after you read each instruction. Take your time and really allow yourself to hear.

1. First, let your hearing focus on individual sounds in your environment.
2. Listen for the sound closest to you.
3. Listen for the sound most distant from you.
4. Listen to the loudest sound.
5. Listen to the quietest sound.
6. Listen to the lowest pitch sound.
7. Listen to the highest pitch sound.

8. Listen for continuous sounds.

9. Listen for cyclical, repeating sounds.

10. Listen for intermittent sounds.

11. Listen through your right ear.

12. Listen through your left ear.

13. Listen through both ears.

14. Now, instead of hearing these sounds one at a time, hear them all at once in a panorama. Listen as if you are broadening your focus from one point on a movie screen to the entire screen. Let go of naming or identifying each individual sound. Hear them combined as one all-encompassing sound. Hold that focus as long as you can.

As you travel through your day, try to take notice of the sounds you ordinarily filter out. Let yourself hear those sounds that surround you all the time that you don't usually hear. Bring into your awareness the qualities of a sound that make it unique: the minute differences and similarities that give it a place in the panoramic auditory spectrum of all the sounds that surround you.

8 ✻ Focusing

There is always music amongst the trees in the garden, but our hearts must be very quiet to hear it.

M. AUMONIER

You are sitting on the sofa in your living room waiting for someone to arrive. It is someone you care about but haven't seen for a while. You hear tires on a driveway, an elevator door, footsteps in the hallway, a key in the lock, or some other sound that lets you know they have arrived. You sit perfectly still and listen. You turn all of your attention to listen for the sound that lets you know they are there. This is focused listening.

We often focus our listening without even noticing. We listen to hear if someone is calling our name, to hear if our child has woken up in the night, to hear wind or thunder in the distance, rain or sleet against our window, or to hear if our car is making a strange noise while we are driving.

When we focus our listening we usually listen for very specific sounds for a short period of time. When we focus our listening for a few seconds, we aren't thinking, just listening. We want to develop, through the practices in this book, our ability to extend the focus of our listening for longer and longer periods of time. By doing so we extend the time between our thoughts.

❀ *Focused Listening Meditation*

1. Close your eyes and listen to one specific sound in your environment.
2. Listen for the subtle fluctuations in pitch, volume, duration, or repetition.
3. Notice when you get distracted and bring your focus back to the sound.

Bill Dixon was a truly innovative composer and trumpet player. His music used timbre, energy, and sonic texture. When instructing players how to play one of his pieces, he would often say, "It's just a sound," meaning, let go of any musical genres or personal musical vocabulary. Let it be unidentifiable as anything other than "pure sound."

❀ *Differentiated Focused Listening Meditation*

1. Pick a piece of music you know that has an individual instrument that plays throughout. Pop, rock, or jazz usually has this quality.
2. Listen through headphones.
3. Focus on just one instrument. Choose the guitar, bass, bass drum, or any instrument that plays a supportive role. Pick something that isn't carrying the main melody.
4. Try to hear its placement in the overall sound, whether it's on the left, right, or in the center of the stereo field. Listen to see if it is in the background or the foreground, the bottom or top of the sound.
5. Listen to that individual part as if it were just playing by itself, as if nothing else were there.
6. See if that individual part makes just one sound or a variety of sounds.
7. Hear its rhythm and how it may change in different parts of the song.

Again, in your daily life, notice what individual sounds you focus on. Try shifting your listening in such a way that you hear things you didn't even know were there.

Also notice that as you focus your listening outward, you are less likely to be talking to yourself, making pictures, or getting feelings. You are less likely to be thinking. If a sound is leading you inward toward thinking, listen to it again and try to hear it as "just a sound" without a name, without a meaning.

9 ✸ Hearing the Room

The things that are invisible to you are often the things that most surround you.

JON HASSELL

ACOUSTICS

Acoustics are the sound qualities of a room. When we hear a sound we also hear the reflection of the sound off of the surfaces of the room. In the same way that light is reflected by a mirror or absorbed by a dull black wall, sound is reflected by hard flat surfaces, such as tile or concrete, and absorbed by soft irregular surfaces like a heavy curtain.

The flat hard tiles of a bathroom reflect sound. They give the room's surfaces a "live," bright, reverberative quality. This is why we all sound so good singing in the shower. In a room that has curtains, a rug, and sound-absorbing ceiling tiles, sound is immediately absorbed. This gives the room a "dead," muffled sound. Recording studios often have sound-absorbing baffles, curtains, and rugs so that the recorded sound isn't colored by the acoustics of the surrounding room.

The size of a room also affects its acoustic qualities. In a small tiled bathroom the sound bounces from one wall to another very quickly. It doesn't have far to travel. Although it does reverberate off the tile, the sound doesn't last very long.

In a large space like a high school gymnasium, the sound has farther to travel before it bounces from the wall to the floor to the ceiling, spreading out around the room. This makes the sound seem to last longer. In large stadiums the reverberation can hang in the air for ten seconds or more after the original sound is made.

If musicians are playing harmonically and rhythmically complex music, the acoustic reflections of the room can build up to make a muddy, unfocused sound. Many new concert halls spend a great deal of money to tune the acoustics of their space. A large cathedral with acoustics of gentle long reflections is a wonderful place for the slow simplicity of Gregorian chant. It's not such a good place for the rhythmic, harmonic complexity of a rock band.

10 ✺ Echolocation

Music is the harmonious voice of creation; an echo of the invisible world.

GIUSEPPE MAZZINI

A dolphin is moving through the water at about twenty-five miles an hour. Although it has keen eyesight, it is unable to see because a recent storm has stirred up fine sand, making the visibility less than a foot. This in no way slows the dolphin down. As it swims it makes a series of clicks and popping sounds. To make them, it uses its nasal sinuses below the blowhole on the top of its head. It projects these sounds through the water where they hit sandbars, coral reefs, sunken ships, fish, and the other dolphins in its pod.

These sounds hit the shapes and surfaces around the dolphin and are reflected, bouncing back to it. Hearing this echo through its teeth and lower jaw, the dolphin's brain makes a three-dimensional picture of the size, shape, and structure of what the clicks are reflecting off of. The dolphin uses sound to navigate, avoid predators, and catch its next meal. The detailed sonic image, produced by echo, helps guide it through the murky water.

This is echolocation. It is used by many sea mammals, as well as bats, as a way to "see" when their eyes are of no use. It is also the underlying mechanism of electronic sonar. It allows us to see the sea bottom, fish, and other boats.

On a boat it is possible to hear the songs of whales, the clicking of dolphins, and the "ping" from the sonar of naval vessels as they are reflected off the hull. 9

We humans also have the ability to use echolocation. The distance between our ears, and the structure and shape of them, help us know what direction a sound is coming from. Our brains detect the millisecond differences between when a sound reaches one ear and then the other. The ridges and grooves on our outer ears give reflections in differences of microseconds. All of this input is processed extremely quickly. It lets us know whether sound is coming from our right or left, front or back, above or below us. This gives us a precise sense of where a sound is coming from.

When a blind person is using a long, white cane, it lets those around them know that the person is blind. It is also a way to ensure that there is nothing in the blind person's path. In addition, they use the cane to make a tapping sound that echoes back to them off of surrounding structures. This helps them echolocate their placement in their immediate environment.

Some of the blind also make clicking sounds with their mouths for echolocation. By recruiting unused parts of the brain's visual cortex, some have been able to develop their sense of "hearing" with what is called "facial vision" to such a high level that they are able to sense the space around them in great detail. Using echolocation in these ways, they are able to rollerblade, play basketball, ride a bike in traffic, and other activities usually requiring eyesight.

✵ Acoustic and Reverberation Meditation

1. Close your eyes, clap your hands, and pause.
2. Listen to the subtlety of how the room affects the sound that bounces back to you.
3. Listen for how long the sound lasts in the room. Large rooms (churches, train stations, warehouses, auditoriums) have longer reverberation times than small rooms.
4. Listen to how the surfaces in the room give the sound presence or muffle it.

5. Rooms with sound-reflective material (tile, cement, wood paneling, glass) are more "live" than rooms with sound-absorbing material (carpet, fabric, curtains, wallpaper, acoustic ceilings), which are "dead."

6. Try to hear the shape of the room.

7. Move within the space and listen for subtle shifts in the sound of the room.

11 ✳ Every Room Has Its Note

Hearing with a divine ear is attained by contemplation of the relationship of space and sound.

YOGA SUTRAS 3.42

RESONANT FREQUENCY

Every room has its own sound, its own note. The pitch of this note depends on the size, shape, and volume of the air in the room. By singing or playing the frequency of a room's note, you can make the air and room itself sympathetically vibrate. This note is what is known as a room's resonant frequency.

The resonant frequency of a room is a subtle but powerful thing. If you are in a large open room and sing the note of the resonant frequency, the reverberation will have more resonance and strength than if you sing an unrelated note.

When an unattended microphone feeds back, its pitch is often related to the resonant frequency of the room. The sound of the room's resonant frequency subtly vibrating is picked up by the mic and amplified through the speakers. This makes the room resonate more strongly, which again is picked up by the mic and fed back into the room. The loop of the room sound, the mic, and the amplification causes volume and harmonics to build into a loud, often shrill tone: feedback.

Resonant frequency was used in 1970 by a pioneering electronic music composer named Alvin Lucier. He composed a piece called "I Am Sitting in a Room." *9* In this piece the performer reads a paragraph that is about a minute and fifteen seconds long and begins with the words, "I am sitting in a room."

As he reads his voice is recorded. That recording is then played back through a set of speakers into the room. As it plays back it is recorded through a microphone on the other side of the room, into another recorder. That second recording is then played back and recorded again on the first machine across the room. This ping-pong process of playback and recording through the air of the room is repeated thirty-two times.

With each successive recording generation, the pitches of the spoken words related to the resonant frequency of the room are amplified by the room itself. Those that are not related fall away. Even after a dozen times you begin to hear just the tone of the words given resonance by the frequency they share with the room. After thirty-two times it's pure sound. It is nothing but a series of swelling tones, the resonant frequencies of the room.

✸ *Resonant Frequency Meditation*

1. Find a nice open, resonant room.
2. Sing or play on an instrument a wide range of different, individual pitches, different high sounds, low sounds, sounds in the middle.
3. See if the sound in the room changes in response to any specific pitches.
4. If you find a particularly resonant pitch, try the pitch right above and below that pitch. Notice if the room responds differently.

12 ✸ I Hear What You're Saying

Before you speak, it is necessary for you to listen, for God speaks in the silence of the heart.

MOTHER TERESA

At the dawn of humanity, prior to language, one of the ways that tribes united and bonded together was through group vocalization. Through chorusing together groups of humans began to give distinct meanings to certain sounds. The evolution of words and language was the natural outcome.

We can see that same evolutionary process compressed into a couple of years as a baby acquires the ability to speak and understand language. Initially a newborn baby hears words as sound without meaning. Only their sound has a physical and emotional impact. As the baby grows older, it starts to learn that specific words have specific meanings. As that happens the qualities of the sound are subjugated to the meaning of the word. It's not that the impact of the sound disappears altogether, it just moves into the background of the unconscious.

The expression "It's not what you said, it's how you said it" is a perfect example. Take the word *Yes*. If we say it softly with a rising inflection at the end, it becomes a question. If we add emphasis on the *y*, lengthen it, and exaggerate the rise, it becomes comic. If we say it loudly with the inflection starting high and dropping, it becomes celebratory.

If we use the same inflection, but drop down low in our range and clip it short, it becomes angry. If we add a quiet breathy quality and lengthen it, the sound becomes plaintive or sensual depending on our range and emphasis in inflection.

There are many auditory components to speech: pitch, volume, rhythm, tempo, and inflection. Often these other components will tell us more about what a person is experiencing internally than the words they are saying.

When we are excited we often speak with a high pitch, at loud volume, with a clipped rhythm, and a fast rate of speed. Conversely, when we are relaxed we tend to speak low in our range, softly, with a more extended rhythm, and at a slower speed.

These are generalizations and don't apply to everyone all the time; nonetheless, individual parts of the sound we are making when we speak can show a great deal above and beyond the content of the words.

THE IDEA OF NORTH

Glenn Gould was a brilliant, eccentric piano virtuoso with formidable technique. He was a child prodigy who could read notes before he could read words. He was best known for his interpretations of Bach's keyboard literature. His recordings were very popular, lauded by many, but criticized by some as being too personally stylized. He was also a composer and conductor.

Gould would often visit a truck stop north of Toronto, where he would listen to the conversations of the customers, not as words with meaning, but just as pure sound. He would listen to the voices in multiple conversations intertwining as if they were the voices of a Bach three-part invention.

This gave rise to a series of radio programs he composed and produced for the Canadian Broadcasting Corporation. In 1967 he assembled an hour-long show, entitled "The Idea of North." 9 It consisted of the voices of five Canadians, men and women, speaking naturally about their experiences of "The North."

The piece was composed and arranged by Gould. The voices were individually recorded. He would then "conduct" the recording engineer as to each voice's entrance, exit, and volume relative to the others as they were mixed into a single recording. He called this style of composition "Contrapuntal Radio." It emphasized the musical interplay of the voices' rhythm, inflection, phrasing, and cadence, as if they were melodies played by instruments. The meaning of the words took a place of lesser importance than their sound. Gould's object was for the listener to hear the voices the same way he heard them, as pure sound.

❀ *Speech as Sound Meditation*

It is best to start in a neutral setting (restaurant, movie theater, or meeting) where a large number of people are all speaking at once.

1. Listen to the sound of their speech rather than their words.
2. Listen to how high or low each voice is pitched.
3. Listen to how loud or soft each voice is speaking.
4. Listen to the length of words and the spaces between them.
5. Listen to how fast or slow each voice is speaking.
6. Listen to how each voice uses inflection to color the intent behind the words.
7. Listen to each voice as if you were listening to a solo instrument playing a melody.
8. Listen to many conversations all at once as one sound.

13 ✵ Body Music

Music melts all the separate parts of our bodies together.

ANAÏS NIN

When I was five years old my family lived in the country where on a quiet summer night you could hear the far-off sound of trains moving through the darkness. As I was falling asleep one night I heard what I thought might be a distant train slowly chugging along. But it seemed different. Even though it was distant it was also inside of my head. The repeated *chug, chug, chug* I heard was a little frightening, but also interesting to me.

The next morning I asked my father about what I had heard. He told me that because of how I had been lying in bed, probably with one of my ears on my arm, I had been able to hear the circulation of my blood as my heart pumped it through my arteries.

There are many sounds our bodies make that we usually don't hear. In the same way we filter out the external sounds that surround us, we filter our internal body sounds. If we didn't there would be so much sound information we would be overwhelmed by what we hear.

To broaden our listening in another way, we will attempt, one at a time, to lift some of these filters that prevent us from hearing the sounds of our body.

Really take your time with this exercise. Take a couple of minutes for each line. Rather than trying to force yourself to hear these sounds, just be relaxed and open to the possibility of hearing them. Mostly, be

49

patient. Remember we have had years and years of practice of not hearing them.

✹ *Body Sounds Meditation*

1. Put your fingers in your ears.
2. Listen for the rumble of your muscle in any movement you make.
3. Listen for the sounds of your mouth: swallowing, tongue and lip movement.
4. Listen to your breath.
5. Listen for the pulse of your heart.
6. Listen for the clatter and grinding of your joints and bones when you move.
7. Listen for the hum of your nervous system.
8. Listen for buzzing or ringing in your ears.
9. Listen to how your body is vibrating.

14 ✺ OM

*Through the sound Om we see the reflection of our own
true nature.*

YOGA SUTRAS 1.27

More than a dozen men wrapped in crimson and yellow robes sit in two
long rows facing one another. On the left, the monk second from the
end raises the back of his straightened right hand toward the left side of
his face, his forearm diagonal across his upper chest. It is a signal that
it is time to begin.

His name is Lobsang. Although he is Tibetan, he has never been to
Tibet. He was born in India where he entered a monastery at the age
of fifteen. He is now is in his forties, though he looks much younger.
He is presently the chant master for the group of monks he is travel-
ing with. The position rotates to a different monk every six months to
avoid attachment to a position of authority.

Lobsang begins to chant an invocation to all Buddhas. He sings a
long phrase by himself, chanting a multi-note chord of sound, the bottom note seemingly lower than humanly possible. *"Oooom ma lue, sem
kun . . ."* He is then joined by the other monks, reciting in unison: *"Ky
gon gur chik. . . ."* A thundering low rhythmic phrase cadences as a high
whistling sound sweeps above it.

The sound is astonishing and beautiful. But for Lobsang and the
other monks this is not a musical experience, it is a spiritual one, a
form of prayer. The ferocity of their multi-phonic chant heightens the

meaning and the action of the ancient sacred text they recite. At the same time, it distorts the pronunciation of the individual words. This obscures its meaning from the idle listener who is not initiated into its deeper tantric meanings.

The transcendent peacefulness on the face of each monk belies the fierceness and fearlessness of their practice and its sound. So engulfed are they in this meditation, the individual self is lost, surrendered to the pure consciousness of the sound. They reach complete union, unaffected by the fluctuations of thought, memory, or the physical body. They become the sound and the sound becomes them. 9

It is no coincidence that most organized religions have some form of singing, chanting, or mantra. When we give sound to the breath, we not only alter our regular breathing patterns but also cause our bodies to vibrate. The breath lengthens and becomes steady, which in turn relaxes and opens both our bodies and our minds. The sound vibration spreads through the body energizing us.

The combination of these two elements helps us be receptive to new ideas, beliefs, and ways of thinking. Making sound together, and synchronizing our breath with others, forms a powerful bond for a group of singers. This is especially true if the sound we make together is beautiful and harmonious.

MANTRA

Mantra derives from two Hindu words *manas* and *tra*. *Manas* means "mind." *Tra* means "protection." The chanting of a sacred mantra protects the mind from idle thoughts and mind chatter. Mantra is an expression of nada yoga.

OM

Om is a sacred sound. It is one of the simplest yet most powerful. It is also one of the oldest and most widely chanted mantras. Om is used by yogis as an invocation at the beginning of practice. It is also used by Hindus, Buddhists, and Jains as an opening, closing, and integral part of many, many chants in all three religions.

✹ *The Outer Om Meditation*

1. Take a nice full inhale.
2. Sing a nice relaxed tone in the lower part of your range.
3. Sing Om for the entire exhale, closing to the *m* at the end of the breath.
4. Let the *m* sound move up into your nose.
5. Repeat this cycle of inhale and exhale until it is effortless and symmetrical.
6. Listen intently to the sound as you make it.
7. Keep your single-pointed attention focused on the sound vibration.
8. Listen to how the sound changes as you move from open, to closed, to nasal sound.
9. Feel where it is vibrating in your body.
10. Let the body become the bow. Let the breath become the arrow. Let the sound of Om become the arrow's point. Let bliss be the target.

Vaikhari

Vaikhari is all the sounds of the world around us. These include natural and mechanical sounds made by man and the sounds we use to communicate: language, vocalization, and music. The more subtle sounds of our ambient environment are acoustics, resonant frequencies, and the internal sounds of our body. Any external sounds we can perceive with our ears are "gross" sounds, the first level of sound, Vaikhari.

PART THREE

Madhyama, the Second Level of Sound

Mind

15 ✸ Outside In

After sounding Om *abandon the vocal sound and dissolve into soundless consonant* m *and into the subtlety of the nada.*

YOGA SUTRAS 1.28

Here are several approaches to mantra that will help us deepen our nada yoga practice.

✸ *The Inner Om Meditation*

1. Sing Om.
2. Sing Om silently to yourself on both the inhale and exhale.
3. Listen to your voice internally, singing Om on the inhale and exhale.
4. Imagine a room full of people singing with you on the inhale and exhale.
5. Hear that Om become continuous, no longer limited by your breath.
6. Hear it rising and falling as individual voices enter and fade out.
7. Imagine the sound of everyone in your town singing Om.
8. Imagine the sound of everyone in your state singing Om.
9. Imagine the sound of everyone in your country singing Om.
10. Imagine the sound of everyone on your continent singing Om.
11. Imagine the sound of everyone in the world singing Om.
12. Hear it quietly connecting back to all the Oms that have ever sounded.
13. Hear it quietly connecting forward to all the Oms that will ever sound.
14. Hear and feel Om vibrating the entire Universe.

SO'HAM

Gorakshanath taught that with every inhale we make the sound *So,* and with every exhale we make the sound *Ham.* Hearing these sounds internally as we inhale and exhale gives our breath an auditory component, So'ham, which we can make a point of attention in meditation. It is an *Ajapa Gyatri,* a silent sacred song.

The sound *So* is Universal Consciousness and *Ham* is our individual consciousness. When you inhale you are drawing in Brahman (the Universal). When you exhale you are releasing the Atman (the Self).

As we are drawn by our breath into a meditative state, our inhale and exhale become slow and soft. As the *So* and *Ham* become indistinguishable, their sound dissolves into a continuous Om. This then is the moment when the sameness of the Universal Consciousness, *So,* and the Divine Self, *Ham,* is revealed as one, Om. "You are that!" the anahata nada.

✸ *So'ham Meditation*

1. As you inhale use your breath to make the sound *So.*
2. As you exhale use your breath to make the sound Ham.
3. Continue to make these sounds as you inhale and exhale for a few moments.
4. Stop making the external sounds as you continue to, internally, hear *So* as you inhale and *Ham* as you exhale for a few moments.
5. Let the consonant *S* on the inhale and *H* on the exhale fall away and continue making the sound *ohh-amm* internally.
6. Let *ohh-amm* shift into an Om that begins with the inhale and continues through to the *mmm* sound at the end of the exhale.

THE FOUR LEVELS OF SOUND

The four levels of sound can be found in the sound of Om: vaikhari in the *O,* madhyama in the *m,* pashyanti in the nasalized *m,* and para in the silence after the sound. The fourth level is a silent echo of the nasalized *m*. It is the transcendent aspect of the sound. In that silence nada will arise.

✸ The Silent Om Meditation

1. Sing Om on the exhale.
2. On the inhale remain silent.
3. Do the same thing internally.
4. Extend the silence between Oms.
5. Leave all sound and dissolve into the silent echo of Om.
6. Listen for the subtlety within the silence.

16 ✸ It's All in Your Mind

Music is the expression of the movement of the waters, the play of curves described by changing breezes.

CLAUDE DEBUSSY

When we perceive something our external sense organs are only a conduit. It is the brain that puts all the pieces together to give us a sense experience. We convert the light entering our eye to electrical impulses that are gathered, sorted, and organized to construct an image.

When we look at a rose we see color, brightness, contrast, shading, outline, perspective, depth of field, movement, and many other gradated attributes. They are each evaluated, many individually, by small localized portions of the brain. Then another portion of the brain takes all the information from these individual parts and constructs the image of a flower.

Our brain uses the same internal neural pathways to recall an image that were used when we originally perceived it. The brain gathers all of the same individual bits of information from small localized areas of memory, where they were stored. It then reconstructs the image. Instead of using the external sense organs for all the individual pieces, they are summoned from our memory. They are then coalesced into an internal image of what we had previously perceived with our senses.

This is also true with the sounds we hear. We distinguish pitch, volume, tone, rhythm, and tempo as individual components and with

59

them reconstruct the totality of a sound. When we recall a sound we gather its individual pieces, then reconstruct them into a whole.

✸ Sound Memories Meditation

1. Remember the sound of a door in your house closing.
2. Remember the sound of your phone ringing.
3. Remember the sound of your car starting.
4. Remember the sound of a dog barking.
5. Remember the sound of laughter from a baby.
6. Remember the sound of surf at the ocean.
7. Remember the sound of a loved one's voice.
8. Remember a special sound from your childhood.

17 ✳ Train of Thought

We may listen to our inner self and still not know which ocean we hear roaring.

MARTIN BUBER

Improvising musicians often hear what they are going to play an instant before they play it. The same is true of singers who hear the pitch they are going to sing before they sing it.

Many of us often hear what we are going to say before we say it. There is a short pause between the formation of these words (madhyama) and our saying them (vaikhari). This gives us an opportunity to decide if we really should say those words or not. We edit and shape what we will say according to changes in the situation or conversation. The stronger the emotion we are about to express, the more difficult it is not to say the words until they are already out of our mouth. Words spoken in anger often have to be taken back later.

✳ Word Formation Meditation

1. Observe how you form a thought and transform it into words.
2. Notice if it starts with a feeling, an image, or another sound.
3. Notice the pause between the formation of the words and speaking them.
4. Notice if, given time, you edit or rewrite the words before saying them.
5. Notice how you adapt words to a changing situation or what others might say.

18 ✹ The Inner Voice

You are just the instrument through which the divine pied piper blows.

VILAYAT INAYAT KHAN

On the morning of September 11th, 2001, at 8:40 a.m., I was parking my car on King Street in Manhattan, about twenty blocks north of the World Trade Center. As I waited for the parking meter to take effect at 9 o'clock, I noticed a group of people standing on the corner looking up and pointing. Then I heard the fire trucks from the firehouse around the corner: Engine 24, Ladder Company 5. They were screaming down Varick Street, the continuous wail of their sirens punctuated by blasts of their horns.

I got out of my car, walked to the corner, and did what everyone else was doing: I looked up. There was a fiery gash in the side of the World Trade Center's North Tower with smoke pouring out of it. I started to walk south toward it. Shortly after crossing Canal Street, I saw an explosion of flames billowing from the South Tower as the second plane hit.

I continued walking south until I reached the corner of Duane Street and West Broadway. This is the neighborhood where I used to live, six blocks north of the Trade Center. Broadway was completely filled with people who had emptied out of the surrounding buildings to see what was happening.

With horror, I watched people jumping to their death.

After almost an hour of helplessly witnessing this horrific tragedy, a voice in my head said forcefully, *It's time to go. Something is going to happen.* I started to walk north back to King Street. Just as I arrived, the first Tower came down.

This is a rather dramatic example of internal dialogue.

On a daily basis many of us have internal dialogue. In the above case it was protective of my survival. It can also be helpful and supportive, making suggestions that aren't in our conscious awareness. It can be encouraging and affirming as we try something at which we are determined to succeed. It can also be self-critical.

We have all had a conversation that didn't go well. We run it over and over in our mind, thinking of other things we could have said. After failing at something we may scold ourselves for our inadequacies.

It is important to understand that underneath all internal dialogue, whether it is a positive affirmation or the tape loops of self-criticism, there is always a positive intent. No matter how harsh or grating the voice might be, it is an expression of a part of us that is trying to take care of us. It is a part that is trying to protect us in some way. It might not be doing it in a way that is helpful at that moment, but there's always an underlying positive intent.

Loving and respecting that part of us that offers these "critical" comments is a big step toward coming to peace with ourselves. It is a way to embrace all of what we are.

✸ *Inner Voice Meditation*

In this meditation we prepare to do the work on our internal dialogue by paying attention to its attributes in our daily life. As you go through your day:

1. Notice when you are having an internal dialogue.
2. Notice the different qualities of the voice you are hearing internally.
3. Listen to the pitch, volume, rhythm, tempo, and inflection.
4. Whose voice is it? Is there more than one voice?
5. Notice any negative loops or self-criticism that may come up.

❀ *Inner Voice Conversation*

When you have a few moments to sit quietly:

1. Engage that critical inner voice in a conversation.
2. Ask the voice what is its positive intent?
3. When you get an answer, thank the voice and lovingly embrace it.
4. Ask it if you can help it find a more appropriate way to accomplish that same positive intent.
5. Play with it by asking it to change its pitch, volume, rhythm, tempo, or inflection.
6. Notice that even when the message remains the same, if the voice is altered, the words have less emotional charge. Taking in the meaning of the message becomes easier.

19 ✸ Picture This

Words form the thread on which we string our experiences.
ALDOUS HUXLEY

Just by reading the words in this book we internally construct intricate and complex visual representations of people, objects, situations, or entire worlds. We are translating combinations of words into pictures and sounds. This is why movies rarely live up to books. The pieces of pictures we make internally are drawn from our memories. The image we create is our own personal version of what has been described in words. The images in a movie are someone else's vision of what the words mean. They can't have the power of images drawn from our own experience.

What an amazing gift to have described to us places we have never been, people we have never met, actions we have never taken, and thoughts we have never had. Our minds combine these bits of memory and sense experiences from our past and bring them to life as an entirely new experience.

✸ Word Pictures Meditation

1. Open a book you have previously read. Pick a passage that is particularly vivid in its visual description.

2. As you read allow yourself to fully enter the internal pictures you make of what is described.

3. Hold the image in your mind and examine what is familiar about it.

4. See if any pieces of what you have fabricated match any of your personal experiences, even if it's just a color or an object.

5. Read the passage a second time. This time allow yourself to witness your process for converting the words into pictures. It happens very quickly. Try to slow it down.

6. Notice if this brings any insight into what sources you are drawing the many individual pieces from to create the totality.

Madhyama

Madhyama is all of our mental sound. This includes sound memories, words we use to form speech, our internal dialogue, and words that paint mental pictures. Madhyama is the internal sounds of the mind.

PART FOUR

Pashyanti, the Third Level of Sound

Visual

20 The Colors of Your Mind

Meditate on the light of the primordial sound between the eyebrows. Join with it in an unbroken stream of luminosity.

Gheranda Samhita 6.17

Visual sounds? How can a sound be visual?

Some genres or schools within an art form are made up of similar artists who share a primary perceptive mode that is different from the sensory mode in which they express themselves.

For a visual artist who primarily takes information in kinesthetically, the feeling of the brushstroke, the gesture, may be of greatest importance in what they express on the canvas. A visual artist who takes in the world through the auditory realm may feel compelled to work with words and text on their canvas.

When sensory input from one sense is perceived as input from a different sense, the experience is called *synesthesia*. In synesthesia what is perceived by one sense is instantaneously converted into an additional internal experience of a different sense. The most common forms of synesthesia are the perception of specific colors as an intrinsic element of specific letters, numbers, musical keys, or notes.

Estimates of the incidence of synesthesia in the general population range from one in twenty-three people to one in eighty. Synesthesia is directly related to some forms of creativity. Neuroscientist Vilayanur S.

Ramachandran says, "Synesthesia is eight times more common among artists, poets, novelists, and other creative people than in the general population."[1] One aspect of creativity is the ability to see connections between disparate objects or ideas.

From birth, as the brain develops both physically and mentally, it divides into separate specialized areas that perform different functions. In synesthetes these walls of separation don't develop between some unrelated areas. The result is that input through one sense may be internally perceived by the brain as the simultaneous blending of two senses. This is how synesthesia naturally occurs. If, while developing, the section of the brain that is responsible for perceiving sound doesn't modularize and instead maintains neural pathways with the parts of the brain that store perception of physical shapes, light, and color, then the sound of the notes of a trombone melody may also be perceived as long, shiny, golden tubes floating through the air.

A sound engineer with synesthesia, while mixing music, may see the stereo image as a panoramic terrain. They place each instrument on the left and right horizontal plane to either differentiate or blend them. They give each its own amount of volume and reverberation to place it in the foreground or distance. They may bring out different parts of its tone quality to give it a sparkling clarity or a shrouded darkness.

A composer who is a synesthete may actually picture the shape of sounds made by different instruments. Notes of melodies may be links of rounded cylindrical bubbles of different lengths. A sustained or drone sound may be a long continuous line like a horizon. Short percussive sounds may be a string of sharp angular shards. The volume of a note may determine its size. Differences in an instrument's sound, the thinness of a flute's notes, as compared to the fatness of the notes of an electric bass guitar, may be reflected in the difference in the shape of the sounds.

To that composer the tone quality of a sound may have a color. How high or low a sound is may determine how high or low it is in this overall visualization. All of these may be part of that composer's way of placing instruments or their sounds in the larger visual picture of an arrangement or orchestration.

Just as the blind person recruits some of the visual brain, some composers who have synesthesia use visual parts of the brain to conceive and compose complex compositions. The many different instruments and the sounds they make are placed in relationship to one another in a visual/aural landscape. Franz Liszt, Nikolai Rimsky-Korsakov, Duke Ellington, Leonard Bernstein, György Ligeti, Stevie Wonder, and Jimi Hendrix are just a few of the composers who were or are synesthetes.

Natural synesthesia is an inherited genetic trait. Even though it only occurs in between one and four percent of people, the potential to cultivate it exists in all of us. We can develop new neural pathways and link otherwise separate sections of our brain, allowing us to see sound.

✳ Musician Visualization Meditation

1. Pick a piece of jazz from the 1950s played by a quartet or quintet (for example, John Coltrane's "Equinox" or Miles Davis's "So What"). ♩

2. Listen to it through headphones.

3. Close your eyes.

4. Imagine you are sitting in a club listening to them play.

5. See the musicians wearing dark suits, ties, and white shirts.

6. Imagine that the club is dark, except where lights are shining on a small raised stage.

7. As you listen pick out the different instruments.

8. As you hear the low throb of the stand-up bass, see the bass player hunched over his instrument as it leans against one shoulder. With his opposite hand he plucks the strings.

9. As you hear the crack and snap of the drums and cymbals, picture the drummer sitting at the back of the stage. His drums are arranged around him, his sticks hit the cymbals and snare drum.

10. As you hear the accompaniment of the piano, see the piano player seated at a grand piano. He moves his hands over the keyboard. His fingers come to rest and press down individual keys.

11. As the trumpet or saxophone plays the melody or improvises, see the musician standing at a microphone at the front of the stage. The horn moves slightly as his fingers raise and lower the valves or keypads.

✾ *Sound Scene Meditation*

1. Choose a dramatic piece of classical music that you don't know (perhaps Debussy's "Sunken Cathedral" ♪ performed by Erich Kunzel and the Cincinnati Pops Orchestra).
2. Listen to it through headphones.
3. Close your eyes.
4. As you hear the music make an internal movie to go with the sound. It can be a landscape, characters moving and interacting, anything that is a visual narrative of what the music is expressing to you.
5. As the music changes allow the story it is telling to unfold as a movie in your mind's eye.

✾ *Sound Texture Meditation*

1. Listen to a piece of purely textural music (for example, Robert Fripp's and Brian Eno's "Wind on Water" or Steve Reich's "Music for 18 Musicians"). ♪
2. Listen to it through headphones.
3. Close your eyes.
4. Visualize a screen on which you can see the music as it is being played.
5. Make an abstract movie of the sound, with shapes, colors, textures, and movement representing the music.
6. As you hear each note visualize what the sound looks like.
7. See high sounds up high on the screen and low sounds down low on the screen.
8. See long notes having long linear shapes. See short sounds having short angular shapes.
9. See loud sounds in the foreground and soft sounds in the background.
10. See different sounds having different colors.
11. See some sounds as shiny and bright and others as dark and dull.

21 ✸ A Soundtrack for Your Life

Music in the soul can be heard by the Universe.

LAO-TZU

In the previous chapter we followed the connection from the world of sound to the visual world. Here we will flow the other way, following the connection of the visual world to the world of sound.

We sometimes refer to someone as having a particular "vibe." In the sixties *vibe* was a colloquial expression for vibration. As I note at the beginning of the book, everything is vibrating, even people. Sounds and sound qualities are ascribed to personality types. We might say that a person is a "crashing bore," "resounding failure," "shrill character," "ringing success," "loud dresser." All these expressions use sound to describe a person's character or how they look.

✸ The Sound of People Meditation

1. As you walk down the street, without judgment, observe people.
2. Imagine that each person has a sound, the sound of their mood, their personality, or the way they move; the sound of their entire being; the sound of their unique vibration. For example, someone might be the sound of a burning fire, a simple melodious tone, electronic static, running water, a pinball machine, or breaking glass.
3. Use your sonic imagination to create a mental sound effects track with a sound for each person you walk by.

✸ *TV Soundtrack Meditation*

1. Watch a show on television that is highly visual (for example, a program on the Travel Channel or Animal Planet).
2. Turn the sound off.
3. Watch the visuals without having to name or identify what you see.
4. Imagine the sounds you would be hearing if you were there.
5. Let yourself feel the mood of the visual (relaxed, active, uplifting, sad, etc.).
6. Imagine a song you know that matches the feeling of the visual.
7. Imagine a song that is the opposite of the feeling of the visuals. Notice how the feeling of the visuals changes.
8. Imagine a musical sound (not a song you have heard before) that would support whatever the visual is. Make it as simple or as complex as you like.

A highly talented musician named Michael Lewis, whom I worked with many years ago, once said to me: "I have music playing in my head all the time. It's like a soundtrack for my life."

✸ *Live Soundtrack Meditation*

1. As you go through your day imagine different music for different activities.
2. At times of activity, or physical movement, hear energetic, rhythmic music.
3. For quiet, relaxed moments, hear slow, melodious music.
4. Try using imagined music to change your mood.
5. If you are rushing and want to relax, imagine slow melodious music.
6. If you are tired and want to motivate yourself, imagine energetic rhythmic music.
7. Notice how specific songs have specific feelings. Just by singing them internally we can shift our mood.

22 ✵ The Lightness of Being

There is a crack in everything, that's how the light gets in.

LEONARD COHEN

Although our primary focus is sound, in the nada yoga meditation, the gateway to that sound is through light. Light and sound are mutually supportive and become woven together as one.

Enlightenment means to "shed light upon." Its attainment is often compared to the lighting of a lamp that shines into the darkness revealing all that surrounds it. That which already exists but is unseen is made visible by the lamp's illumination. Its light makes the unmanifest manifest.

The sacred texts of all major religions contain references to light: luminous, bright, shining, effulgent, illuminating, radiant, lustrous, brilliant, glowing, blazing, fiery light. These sometimes refer to the "light of knowledge" or the "flashing forth of insight," rather than literal light. Most, however, describe people who, while having a transcendent experience, see or are enveloped in a bright radiant light. Visions of saints, angels, or gods are often surrounded by brilliant or fiery light. Illumination and luminance are words equated with transcendent states of higher consciousness.

Many ascendant yogis speak of seeing a bright white light inside or at the crown of the head. Others refer to the "Blue Pearl," an iridescent point of light surrounded by a saffron aurora seen by fixing the gaze between the eyebrows.

Some yogic masters are able to see light within the subtle body, prana moving through the *nadis* (inner channels) as streams of light, the *chakras* (energy centers) emanating different colors of light, the *sushumna,* a cable of radiant light running from the *muladhara* chakra at the base of the spine to the *sahasrara* chakra at the crown of the head.

Those who have had near-death experiences report encounters with a primal, radiant white light. This occurs as the consciousness is leaving the body. This "clear light," as it is described in the *Tibetan Book of the Dead,* is all encompassing and overpowering.

There are tantric practices to transform the body from flesh into light, to transcend the impermanence of the physical vessel by changing it into a body of pure eternal luminescence. If attained, this transmutation gives the yogi the powers that light possesses: mobility to travel through the cosmos, transmission of life-giving energy, and immortality.

Light is omnipresent in our everyday lives. In Vedanta the more pervasive something is, the more subtle it is. The more subtle something is, the more pervasive it is. Our environment is suffused with light. We are surrounded by it, our mood affected by it, our very lives dependent on it. The sun provides us with a medium for our vision as well as life-sustaining energy. Often we miss the pervasive subtlety of light, only noticing it at its extremes, when it is blazingly bright or when it is absent.

Just as sound is absorbed and reflected, so is light. Shiny, glossy, mirror-like surfaces reflect light directly. Dull, soft, textured surfaces absorb light. Light refracted through crystal, water, and cut glass divides into the colors of the spectrum. These subtle differences are around us all the time.

✸ Everything Is Illuminated Meditation

1. Observe the different sources of light in your environment.
2. Observe where there is direct light.
3. Observe where there is reflected light.
4. Observe where there is shadow.
5. Observe where there is darkness.

6. Observe the gradation between darkness and light.
7. Observe any refraction as light reflects off of or passes through objects.
8. Observe different hues in visible light.
9. Observe any luminescence or dullness of different colors.
10. Observe how different light sources interact.
11. Observe how some objects or people appear luminescent.

Pashyanti

Pashyanti is the third level of sound, visual sound. It is similar to synesthesia. An external sensory input in one modality that is internally perceived in another sensory modality is synesthesia. A synethete might see sounds or hear colors. This is an ability that can be cultivated over time. At first we use imagination to generate visuals to accompany sound or sound to accompany visuals. Eventually we cultivate the skill to internally represent sensory input in alternative ways. This will be helpful as we move into the meditations on internal light and sound.

PART FIVE

Para, the Fourth Level of Sound

Beyond

23 ✺ Infinity and Beyond

Reabsorption goes beyond sound. Without sound there is no space, only the Ultimate Reality.

HATHA YOGA PRADIPIKA 4.101

Para means "beyond," beyond what the organs of the senses perceive, beyond what can be seen by the eye, beyond what can be heard by the ear, beyond the external to the internal: to arrive, first, at the Divine Light, and then the Sacred Sounds.

Anahata, the unstruck sound, also describes the nada. It is like the vibration of a bell after it has been struck. But, there is no need to strike it to begin the sound, no need to re-strike it to prevent the sound from fading away. It's just there: sustained, continuous, without beginning or end. It is the unchanging constant of Universal Consciousness that exists within each of us. By perceiving and following it we drop into deeper levels of meditation and rise to higher states of consciousness.

There are six meditations in this section. They are progressive, each one interlocking with and building on the previous meditation. Allow yourself time to become fully familiar with each one before moving to the next. You should be able to do the steps of each meditation without having to refer to the book. Then, when you move to the next meditation, the previous one will automatically be available. At that point you can focus on absorbing the new information.

When you have thoroughly learned all of the steps and put them together, they will compress into one automatic process that requires no thinking. Like the individual pieces of a puzzle, they will fall into place forming a larger unified whole.

24 ✷ The Six Pieces

When the yogi is absorbed in the nada, the external world falls away and bliss arises.

SHIVA SAMHITA 5.45

In this section we will go step by step through the daily practice of nada yoga.

1. Posture
2. Unconditional Love
3. The Light
4. Absorption with the Light
5. The Sound
6. Absorption with the Light and Sound

The first step is learning how to sit while we meditate. The next step is finding unconditional love in our heart. Next is the visual aspect of the meditation, how and where to focus our eyes, a description of the internal light and where it will appear. This is followed by how to co-absorb with the light. Then we focus on the sound of the nada, how and where to listen, what we will hear, and how to co-absorb with the sound. Finally, we will integrate the light and the sound; the result is bliss.

It should be emphasized here that, initially, strong effort must be taken to concentrate on seeing the light and hearing the sound. The effort must be in attention, not in an attempt to make something happen. The effort must be in sustaining, with a loving heart, the active looking and focused listening, rather than trying to make light or sound appear. After practicing for some time the mind becomes quiet. Then the effort of attention is replaced by awareness. Rather than actively trying to focus our attention, we are simply witnessing our internal perceptions.

It is important to discriminate between what we imagine and what we internally perceive. It is important to recognize the difference between the sights, sounds, and feelings we create and those we witness. When someone reads us a story the images and sounds we experience are generated by our imagination. With this meditation the light and the sound are internal perceptions. They aren't imagined. They aren't a memory or fantasy. They are as real as what we see and hear in the external world.

25 ❋ The Posture

When there is stillness in body and mind, indescribable
bliss arises.

HATHA YOGA PRADIPIKA 4.32

HOW TO SIT

If you can sit in *siddhasana* that is ideal. To do so, place the left heel
in the middle of the perineum (fig. 1). Place the right heel above the
pubic bone (fig. 2) and roll the right knee down (fig. 3). Tuck the toes

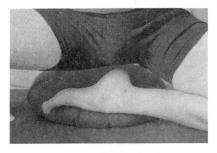

1. Left heel under perineum

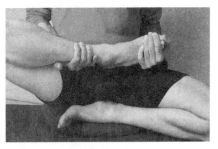

2. Right heel above pubic bone

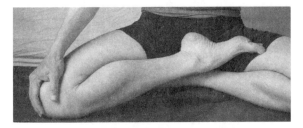

3. Roll right knee down

of the right foot into the fold between the bottom of the left thigh and the top of the left calf (fig. 4). Bring the toes on your left foot up between the thigh and calf on the right leg (fig. 5). Place your hands, palms down, on your knees with your arms straight (fig. 6). This will keep your spine straight.

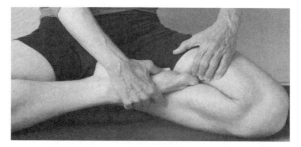

4. Tuck right toes

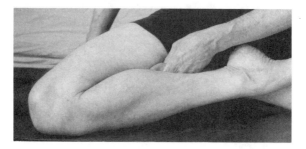

5. Bring up left toes

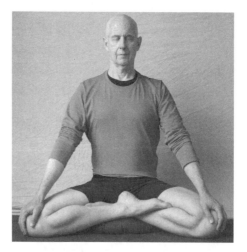

6. Hands on knees, straight arms

If this is not possible, sit on a rolled up blanket or pillow pointed back to front with your legs folded on both sides of it. The blanket or pillow should put pressure on your perineum. Sit comfortably with your body in symmetry. Let the right side of your body (hands/arms, feet/legs) be in the same position as the left side. Place your hands, palms down, on your knees with your arms straight.

The *Yoga Sutras* say "Sthira sukham asanam." This is instruction on the elements of posture when meditating. In Monier Williams' Sanskrit-English dictionary one definition of *sthira* is "still." *Sukha* literally means "a good axle hole," one that is properly centered in the hub so that the wheel isn't out of kilter. This makes for a comfortable ride. *Asana* means "sitting" or "seat"; therefore, "Sthira sukham asanam" instructs us to sit in comfortable stillness.

Once you have found a comfortable way to sit, remain perfectly still. This will facilitate the emergence of a blissful state.

Why do we sit perfectly still?

YOGA NIDRA

There is a well-known image of the cosmos as an ocean. On that ocean is floating a snake. Reclining on the snake is Vishnu. He sleeps and dreams the Universe into existence. It manifests as a lotus flower growing out of his navel. Vishnu's sleep is the sleep of the yogi, *yoga nidra*.

In T. K. V. Desikachar's commentary on Sankara's poem, the *Yoga Taravali,* yoga nidra is described as, "where the person is so strongly linked to the Atman [Divine Self/Universal Consciousness] that he or she is oblivious to all else. So, for an outsider, it seems as if the person is sleeping even though he/she is very much awake. . . ."[1]

Joseph Campbell says, "In deep dreamless sleep consciousness is still there, but it is covered over by darkness. But, suppose you could find that consciousness. Suppose you could go into deep sleep AWAKE!"[2]

Yoga nidra is the ability to keep the mind awake, aware, and in single-pointed focus while inducing the body to sleep. How do we do that?

THE FOUR STATES OF CONSCIOUSNESS

The *Mandukya Upanishad* and the *Shiva Sutras* tell us there are four aspects of consciousness: waking, dreaming, deep sleep, and Universal Consciousness.

In waking consciousness we use our organs of perception to experience the external world. In the dream state we perceive our internal world through mental activity. In deep sleep there is no activity. Universal Consciousness, the fourth state, is present in all three of these states—there is no external perception or internal perception, but neither is there unconsciousness. There is only Consciousness.

The state of waking consciousness is the largest part of our experience. It is our daily life.

When we sleep we go through cycles of the first three states of consciousness. In a night most people have three to six cycles of deep sleep, dreaming, and brief periods of waking. To reach Universal Consciousness we must journey, awake, first through dreaming, then through deep sleep.

The dream state is also called REM (Rapid Eye Movement) sleep, which occurs when we dream. If we can bring the body into REM sleep, while keeping the mind awake, alert, but without mental activity, this is our doorway to deep sleep while still awake. Eventually this can lead us to Universal Consciousness.

How do we take this first step? How do we bring the body into sleep and keep the mind awake? The answer is physical stillness.

ATONIA

In REM sleep our body experiences *atonia,* sometimes referred to as sleep paralysis. It is what keeps us perfectly still while dreaming. If we were able to move, we might physically react to what we are experiencing in our dreams and injure ourselves. In the textbook *Neuroscience: Exploring the Brain,* the authors describe how "[t]he same core brain stem systems that control the sleep process of the forebrain also actively inhibit our spinal motor neurons preventing the descending motor activity from expressing itself as actual movement."[3]

For anyone who has woken up in this state, not knowing that it was atonia, it can be a frightening experience. But if we enter it willingly, rather than feeling held in an immobilizing constriction, we experience a deep feeling of comfort. We feel so good we hold perfectly still in order not to lose that feeling.

Have you ever taken a light nap and felt totally comfortable? If you then moved your arm or leg you may have found you were unable to reenter that feeling of deep comfort, even if you put your limbs back in the exact same position. It's because you were transitioning out of atonia. Our body learns that if we move, we will lose that feeling of deep comfort. As a result we stay perfectly still. Perhaps it is the inhibition of our motor neurons that causes this feeling of comfort.

We know in the nervous system that what is *cause* and what is *effect* are sometimes interchangeable. When we are deeply relaxed our breathing is slow, soft, and regular. Yogis millennia ago discovered that by making their breath slow, deep, and regular, they could induce a feeling of deep relaxation. What flows one way, flows the other.

They also discovered that by staying perfectly still they could experience the deep comfort or bliss of atonia. This feeling, usually experienced when unconscious in sleep, could then be experienced while awake and conscious. The mind is awake while the body is asleep: yoga nidra. Remaining perfectly still is the secret of how to ascend to this seat of bliss.

Falling asleep takes about twenty minutes. So give yourself plenty of time for this next meditation.

✸ Sitting Meditation

1. Sit in siddhasana or sit on a blanket or pillow with pressure on your perineum.
2. Put your hands on your knees.

3. Keep your spine straight.

4. Close your eyes.

5. Let the body relax.

6. Keep the mind alert.

7. Sit comfortably in complete stillness.

8. Notice where discomfort or the need to move arises.

9. Acknowledge it and come back to conscious stillness.

26 ✺ All You Need Is Love

Turn the mind's eye to the point within the heart where the light of the Divine Self burns.

ADVAYA TARAKA UPANISHAD 10

THE POWER OF UNCONDITIONAL LOVE

We are born with an infinite capacity for unconditional love, a love without desire, possessiveness, or the expectation of anything in return. We are born with the light of love shining in our hearts, emanating outward. We are born with the vibration of love sounding deep in our hearts.

You can see the love in the eyes of a baby looking into their mother's face. Even before a child can speak, you can hear the love in the sounds they make looking into their mother's eyes.

As we grow up and live our lives we experience injuries, wounds, and insults to our body, psyche, and spirit. Rejection, humiliation, loss, and other trauma create emotional scars. These scars accumulate over time forming an emotional shell around our heart. This shell becomes thick, a hard callous to protect us from further suffering, pain, and sadness.

Even under the thickest of shells, the divine light of love still shines in our hearts; it has just been covered over. The sacred sound of love still vibrates in us, it has just become muted.

Even though we may become completely numb, within all of us

there still exists the infinite capacity for unconditional love. Look at the face of the mother looking at her newborn child and you will see it.

Unless we have been subjected to the most extreme deprivation, we have all experienced what it is to feel unconditional love. Although it may have happened before we were old enough to be consciously aware of it, we have all experienced unconditional love toward someone or something. If we are a parent, we may have felt it toward our child. We may have felt it toward a pet. We may have felt it toward a place, or something as general as a beautiful day in nature.

We carry the capacity for unconditional love within us everywhere we go, at all times. All we need to do is remember a time when we experienced it, and bring that feeling into the present moment in our life.

It is possible, over time, to dissolve the shell around our heart by letting the light of love shine and the sound of love vibrate, even if it's only for an instant. By experiencing unconditional love we begin the process of dissolving the scars that form that shell.

Every time we put unconditional love into action toward someone else, we let that light burn away the shell and shine on them. Every time we act with kindness, love, or compassion in our daily life, no matter how small the act, we are emanating a vibration that dissolves the shell and spreads sympathetically to vibrate in those around us.

It can be scary at first, feeling so vulnerable, opening ourselves up to the possibility of rejection and pain. Over time we discover that, not only does it make the people around us feel good, but we feel so much better ourselves.

There is no doubt that love conquers every fear. The next time you're feeling fearful about something small, just take a moment to let unconditional love surface in your heart. Amazingly, the fear will disappear.

This is where the impulse that leads to acts of heroism comes from. It is a moment of unconditional love that surfaces in an emergency situation. A person, without even thinking about it, puts someone else's life or well-being ahead of their own. We all have that potential within us.

✸ *Unconditional Love Meditation*

1. Recall a time when you felt unconditional love for someone or something.
2. Remember the place.
3. Remember what you were seeing.
4. Remember what you were hearing.
5. Feel the love as fully as you can.
6. Let your entire attention rest on that love in your heart.
7. Let that feeling of love grow and expand, filling your entire body and mind.
8. Let that feeling of love radiate outward from you, filling the space around you.

27 ✸ The Light

Fixing the pupils on the light causes samadhi.

HATHA YOGA PRADIPIKA 4.39

This is the visual aspect of the nada practice. In the same way visual sounds were discussed in part four, "Pashyanti, the Third Level of Sound," we will find, as we progress through the practice, the intertwining of the internal light and the internal sound. The light is the environment, the internal landscape. The sound is the internal guide that leads us to higher realms of consciousness.

FIXING OUR GAZE

Close your eyes. By closing your eyes and focusing internally you have turned your vision away from the visual stimulation of the outside world. You turn your perception of light inward from your organs of perception, your eyes, to your internal world.

Look up between your eyebrows through closed eyelids. Although you are actively looking/watching, try to make this effortless, without strain. You will eventually see an internal light.

YOGA NIDRA

Here again we see a correlation between entering the REM state and entering yoga nidra.

In everyday life when we close our eyes we stop the flow of visual information to the brain. We automatically shut down the visual cortex, the portion of the brain that processes visual information.

When we enter REM sleep the visual cortex comes back to life. In the REM state the visual cortex is just as active as it is when we are awake with our eyes open. In this meditation we bring the body to stillness. Then, after shutting our eyelids, if we actively *look* with our eyes, we reengage the visual cortex in much the same way it is active in REM sleep. The mind is awake while the body is asleep: yoga nidra.

WHAT WE SEE

At first you may see only darkness. You may see light right away or it may take some time. Eventually you will begin to see flickering lights, clouds of light, rays of light, or colors. When you do begin to see light, it is not imagined. It is an internal perception. This internal light is described in various commentaries on the *Yoga Sutras*:

Swami Satchidananda calls it ". . . a brilliant divine light, which is beyond all anxieties, fear and worry—a supreme Light in you."[1]

Georg Feuerstein quotes the *Mahanarayana Upanishad,* which calls it ". . . a minute, fiery flame, rising up radiant. . . ."[2]

B. K. S Iyengar refers to the glowing of "the sorrowless, effulgent light."[3]

Jyotsna of Brahmananda says the light is "the source of all . . . the supreme *Reality*."[4]

Swami Hariharananda Aranya speaks of, "the effulgent centre of the head."[5]

Swami Kuvalayananda's translation describes it as "Ultimate *Reality*," that which "illuminates everything."[6]

Initially you may only see short flashes of light. The joy you feel in making contact may disrupt that contact. When you start seeing an internal light for longer periods of time, thoughts may come up and distract you.

When they do, notice them, and then bring yourself back to actively looking at the light.

Even if you do not see the light, keep your eyes focused between your eyebrows. Cultivate concentration in spite of momentary breaks between you and your point of focus.

Think of the moments of quiet concentration as spaces between your thoughts. Draft off of these silent spaces like a cyclist drafts off of a rider in front of them. Let yourself be effortlessly pulled along in that silent gap, extending little by little your internal focus on the light.

Once again we see the similarities between REM sleep and yoga nidra. In the prefrontal cortex, which is responsible for thinking and decision-making, there is very little activity during REM sleep. Accessing that state, while coming to single-pointed focus, we bring the mind to stillness.

The next step is for our focus on the light to come to steadiness, our attention uninterrupted by distractions. With continuous unbroken concentration, the nature of the light changes. As we hold our gaze and mind in stillness, the flickering will eventually become a single focused point of light. It may be a fleck of light, a very small, intense dot of light, an iridescent blue or indigo "pearl" surrounded by a saffron-colored corona, a bright burning ball of white light, a star of shimmering light, or other concentrations of brilliant radiance.

In *The Philosophy of Gorakhnath,* Akshaya Kumar Banerjea writes "Gorakhnath advises a yogi to concentrate his attention upon *Nila-Jyoti* (blue self-luminous light) at the inner centre of the eyes. Deep concentration of the whole consciousness upon this *Jyoti* would gradually lead to the spiritual illumination of the consciousness and spiritualisation of his being."[7]

✸ Internal Light Meditation

1. Close your eyes.
2. Look up between your eyebrows.
3. Make this effortless, without strain.
4. Watch for flickering light or clouds of colored light.
5. Steadily concentrate on the light until it becomes a single, focused point.

28 ✹ Absorption

There is no other absorption which equals the Nada.
HATHA YOGA PRADIPIKA 1.43

Eventually you, your focus on the light, and the light will all merge into one. Although the light is a connection to the greater Universe, it is a part of you. By recognizing that connection you become one with the greater Universe.

How do we do that? How do we merge ourselves with the looking and what we are looking at: the light?

There is a phrase that comes from Vedanta, "Tat tvam asi." "You are that!" "You" is the *jivatma* in you. Jivatma is both the individualized ego and the Divine Self. The ego is hiding or covering the Divine Self. "That" is Brahman, which is Universal Consciousness, eternal, unchanging, and that which enlivens everything. "You are that!" is the moment of realization that our Divine Self, stripped of the veil of ego, is the same as Universal Consciousness. They are one.

Clay is molded into many shapes: bowls, pots, cups, and pitchers. They are all pieces of pottery, all individual, and all different. But, they are all, at their essence, still clay. The clay of Brahman is given form in the pottery of the Atman, the Divine Self.

Atman and Universal Consciousness are the same. If we recognize the Divine Self within us all, we recognize the divine nature of Universal Consciousness. This recognition is the realization "Tat tvam asi!" "You are that!"

When you have come to a point where nothing exists but your focus and the light, you can lovingly draw together with it, surrender to it, embrace it, and merge with it. Since the light is within us, it is possible to become enveloped by it and become one with it.

Even though it is internal the light may seem to be hanging in front of and above you. Realize that you are not separate from the light. Truly know "you are that." Draw the light to you. At the same time draw your eyes back in toward the center of your head, pulling the light with them. Dissolve into the light as it dissolves into you.

You may feel the light as well as see it. Feel as if you are *moving forward* as the light spreads out over the front of your head. Wrap it around the top of your head, shoulders, waist, arms, sides, all the way around to your back. Feel the bliss as you become one with it. Continue the slight feeling of moving forward into the light to maintain the co-absorption.

Realize that you always have been, and always will be, one with the light. As you feel it surround and embrace you, flowing over your head and body, let yourself be carried by the bliss as if you were riding it.

✳ *Light Absorption Meditation*

1. Look up between your eyebrows. Make this effortless, without strain.
2. Watch for flickering lights, clouds or rays of light, or colors.
3. If light arises, steadily concentrate on it until, over time, it becomes a single, focused point.
4. Co-absorb with the light by moving it into the center of your head.
5. As you do so pull your eyes back in toward the center of your head.
6. Let the light spread over your head and around your body.
7. Continue moving forward into the light.

As we deeply dissolve with the inner light, we may have the feeling of a physical space surrounding us. Space is often described as the fifth element, *akasha,* empty radiant space. Akasha is inseparably intertwined with sound. Where there is akasha (space), there is sound. Where there is sound, there must be akasha.

29 ✳ The Sound

*Indescribable bliss arises in the heart of the yogi who
meditates on the nada.*

HATHA YOGA PRADIPIKA 4.81

As we turn toward hearing the Inner Sacred Sound, we hold our co-
absorption with the light. We hold that open space in which our mind
and the light are one. When we are steadily in this space, we add to our
attention, listening for sound.

There is a nadi, a subtle nerve channel, that starts under the right
eye. It runs down the cheek, to the jawbone, along the jawline to its
hinge and onto the neck. There it runs back up behind the right ear.
To help find this nadi, trace its path with your right index finger.

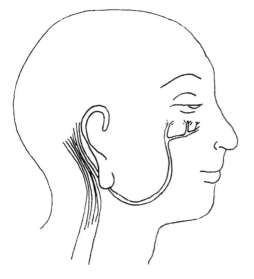

*Trace the path of this nadi
to help connect the light and
sound.*

Awareness of this channel will help you connect the light and sound.

The sound is an internal sound. It is a very subtle sound. If you don't hear it right away, be patient. Attentively wait with unconditional love and a joyful anticipation for the sound to arise. Allow for the possibility that in time you will hear it. All the while maintain your co-absorption with the light.

HOW TO FOCUS YOUR LISTENING

Close both of your ears by physically blocking them. You can use your fingers but this will cause a sound of its own that may be distracting. Foam earplugs, which you can buy at any drugstore, are the best way to seal the ears without creating other sound. They are the best way to turn your perception of sound inward.

When you have been practicing for a while, you will not need to physically close your ears. Through mental constraint you will be able to concentrate on the internal sound to the exclusion of external sounds around you.

Concentrate on the subtler than subtle sound. As some sounds become obvious, continue to seek the most subtle aspect of the sound.

This takes intense focus. Strive to listen to all aspects and frequencies of the internal sound. Find the most subtle part of the sound: the sound behind, above, within, or beyond the sound. Through deliberate and sustained concentration, fix your attention on that part.

You may hear several sounds at once. Some will become pronounced. Some will be more subtle. Focus on the sound that is highest in pitch and has a sparkling iridescence. This is the Inner Sacred Sound.

Finding the most subtle sound calls for a comparison of different sounds. We concentrate on one sound, engage the mind in evaluation, then concentrate on the next and compare the two. This takes concerted concentration.

If you are hearing the internal sound and your mind wanders, bring yourself back to focused listening. The most obvious indication that you have lost contact with the internal sound is if you begin talking to yourself. *If you are listening, you can't be talking to yourself. If you are talking to yourself, you can't be listening.* When you do start talking to yourself, recognize it as a cue to go back to focused listening.

Like extending the length of our focused listening in the external world (see chapter 8), we want to cultivate longer periods of uninterrupted internally focused listening. As you listen with greater and greater focus to the nada, and your concentration becomes unbroken, your internal dialogue stops.

Initially when you are able to sustain concentration, you may feel a certain joy of accomplishment and congratulate yourself on being able to do so. This commenting breaks the continuity of the flow of concentration. Just notice that this has happened, have a little laugh, then return to focused listening. Over time the periods of uninterrupted flow without self-comment will become longer and longer. Your mind will become steadily fixed on the sound in an unbroken stream of concentration without other mental activity. Whatever sound the mind is drawn to, settle on it, adhere to it, and become absorbed in it.

WHAT TO LISTEN FOR

The first sounds you hear may be loud. As your practice grows and your ability to focus increases, you will begin to hear the subtler aspects of sound.

The sound may take many forms: a low rumble; a high, sustained tone; a shimmering vibration; a resonant ringing; or buzzing. The lower sounds are those usually heard first and are sometimes felt in the body as well as heard in the head. Then comes the midrange sounds that are more resonant. The higher sounds have a sparkling, modulating, luminescent quality.

You may also feel a tingling above the soft palate. Gorakshanath describes this location, the root of the palate, as the *talu* chakra. He says it is the tenth door that leads upward to the divine.

Initially it is best not to get attached to one particular sound. The sounds you hear may change from day to day, from meditation to meditation. It is the concentration on these internal sounds that is most important, rather than which sound we hear on any given day. Ultimately, after regular steady practice, your concentration will settle on the highest, most luminous sound.

The *Hatha Yoga Pradipika* lists external sounds that are similar to those that may be experienced internally: ". . . the ocean, thunder, a large waterfall, low drums, large bell, conch shell, horn, flute, tinkling chimes, bees or crickets." ♪

In contemporary terms the instrument most like the nada's high sustained sound is a single note of guitar feedback. As it rises through the harmonics bringing out different shimmering subtleties, it is strikingly similar to the nada. There is also a similarity to overtone singing. Much like the nada, there is a subtlety to each of the individual pitches that make up the harmonic series of overtone singing. ♪

We must learn to discriminate between the sounds of our own body: our breath, blood pumping, or the electrical energy of the nerves and the other deeper sounds behind the audible sound, the nada. This is true even in the case of tinnitus.

TINNITUS

Tinnitus is defined by many as the perception of sound when there is none in the external environment. Strangely enough this is the exact definition some might give to the Inner Sacred Sound of the nada.

There are two schools of thought about tinnitus. One point of view is what most doctors will tell you: it is an incurable disease that afflicts millions of people. As you grow older it becomes more pronounced.

The other point of view is that it is the first stage of hearing the nada. Shri Brahmananda Sarasvati said about tinnitus: "This inner sound, then, is . . . coming . . . from heaven, through our body and mind to alert us to pay attention to our inner life. . . . It is the inner manifestation of a grace, not a curse."[1]

Although tinnitus is a slight obstacle, it isn't the most subtle aspect of the internal sound. If you have it, it is a possible place to begin, but listen for an even subtler sound. When your concentration is completely focused, you won't hear the tinnitus. Your attention will only be focused on the sound of the nada.

WHERE TO FOCUS YOUR LISTENING

The *Hatha Yoga Pradipika* tells us to "listen with one-pointedness to the sound of the nada within the right ear."

Why must we only listen through the right ear? What is perceived by the right ear is processed by the left brain. The left brain is also where the center that processes speech formulation is located. By focusing our listening attention specifically on where speech is formed, we override our ability to make words. If we attentively focus our listening there, we can't be talking to ourselves. We quiet the mind.

ABSORPTION INTO THE SOUND

Empty of internal thoughts and external distractions, focus your listening so that you hear nothing but the nada without interruption. Pull the sound from your right ear, into and around yourself. Let the sound pour into your head and your body as if you were a pot filling with water. Let the sound vibrate everywhere inside of you. Put yourself in the sound and the sound in your Self. Become the sound and let the sound become you. Feel the connection between your vibration and the vibration of the greater Universe. Know that they have always been, and will always be, the same.

✸ *Internal Sound Meditation*

1. Close your eyes.
2. Mentally trace the subtle nerve channel that runs from below the right eye to behind the right ear.
3. Listen for sound within your right ear.
4. Listen for the most subtle part of the sound. It will get louder.
5. Pull the sound from your ear into yourself, filling your head and body.
6. Dissolve into the sound.

30 ✸ Absorption into Light and Sound

The mind redissolves into the Inner Sacred Sound and the Internal Divine Light, and they are again recognized as one.

HATHA YOGA PRADIPIKA 4.100

If you can hold two points of attention at once, it is impossible to have an internal dialogue. Our two points of attention are active looking and focused listening. If we hold both, we can't be talking to ourselves. This inner quiet then opens the way for deeper levels of meditation.

Hold the space in which you have dissolved into the light and dissolved into the sound. When you are able to concentrate on both the sound and light and they are both evident, they support and amplify one another. As the sound gets louder absorption into the feeling of the light deepens. As your cohesion with the light becomes stronger, the nada becomes louder. Realize that they are manifestations of the same thing. They are one. You are part of that one. Draw them into and around you. Merge with them. Blend the mind with the Inner Sacred Sound and Internal Divine Light. Blissfully feel them surrounding you, embracing you. Become one with them. Dissolve into them. Let that blissful feeling flow over and through your body.

Para

Para is the fourth level of sound. Para is beyond. To go beyond we go within. We go beyond ourselves by going within ourselves. We go beyond how we usually sit into sitting in complete stillness. We go beyond our day-to-day self by holding unconditional love in our hearts. We go beyond what our eyes can see in the external world by looking within and seeing the Internal Divine Light. We go beyond what our ears can hear by listening within the sound within us and hearing the Inner Sacred Sound. We go beyond our self by going within our Self and realizing it is one and the same as Universal Consciousness. Para, going beyond, is an infinite expansion.

PART SIX

The Practice

31 ✸ The Four Components

*When the light of Universal Consciousness shines forth and
removes ignorance, the yogi perceives Reality without the
play of the world.*

YOGA TARAVALI 27

Now we have the four basic components of the meditation: stillness in
posture, unconditional love, absorption with the Internal Divine Light,
and absorption with the Inner Sacred Sound.

Stillness is the solid ground on which to build the foundation of
this meditation. Unconditional love is the vessel in which Internal
Divine Light and Inner Sacred Sound are nurtured and cultivated. If
rather than trying to make the light and sound appear we invite them
to come, with that feeling of unconditional love in our hearts, they are
more likely to arise. If we surrender to that feeling of love, they're more
likely to re-unite with us, letting us fully experience bliss. Trust that we
already know how to do all of this.

In the next two chapters the basic meditation will be presented in
two forms: the first, with full in-depth instructions; the second, with
simple one-line instructions. The repetition and condensation of the
instructions in chapters 32 and 33 are to promote self-practice. This
progression is to encourage you, in meditation, to further simplify the
instruction. With practice you will only need a single phrase or word to
trigger a part of the meditation that took an entire chapter to explain.

32 ✸ The Basic Meditation with Full Instructions

Meditation on the blissful light within brings the mind to stillness.

YOGA SUTRAS 1.36

1. Sit comfortably with your body in symmetry. Let the right side of your body (hands/arms, feet/legs) be in the same position as the left side. If you can sit with your legs crossed with one of your heels pressing up into your perineum, that is ideal. If not, sit on a rolled up blanket or pillow placed longways between your legs so there is pressure on your perineum.
2. Block the sound entering your ears with earplugs. You can use your fingers instead, although this will cause a sound of its own, which may be distracting.
3. Put your hands on your knees. This will prevent you from slumping. Keep your spine straight. (If your fingers are in your ears, sit with your feet flat on the ground and your knees up. Put your elbows on your knees.)
4. Close your eyes.
5. Try to find a position of comfort so you don't have to move. You want to be able to sit in perfect stillness for yoga nidra to arise.
6. Recall a past experience of unconditional love. Fill your heart with that feeling. Repose in the center of your heart, suffused with that unconditional love.

7. With your eyes still closed, look up between your eyebrows. Your gaze is inward, but your focus is as if you were looking outward into the distance. Although you are actively looking/watching, try to make this effortless, without strain.

8. With a feeling of unconditional love and sense of joyful anticipation, invite the Divine Light to arise.

9. Allowing the light to arise is something we intuitively and naturally know how to do. The light is already shining within us. With unconditional love, surrender your control over it.

10. Quiet your mind. Let go of all thinking. If thoughts come up, let them pass like a cloud in the sky. Then bring your focus back to looking/watching between your eyebrows.

11. At first you may see only darkness. Eventually you will begin to see flickering, clouds or rays of color, or lights. These are not imagined. They are an internal perception.

12. If light arises, hold it in your attention without trying to control it. Thank it with unconditional love for arising. With continuous unbroken concentration, over time, the lights will eventually become a single focused point of light. It may be a very small, intense dot or fleck of light, an iridescent blue or indigo "pearl" surrounded by a corona, a bright burning ball of white light, a shimmering star, or other concentrations of brilliant radiance.

13. Realize that you are not separate from the light. Embrace that "You are that." Co-absorb with the light by moving it into the center of your head.

14. At the same time, draw your eyes back in toward the center of your head, pulling the light with them.

15. Draw the light into and around you. As you dissolve into it and it into you, blissfully feel it surrounding and covering your head. Let that blissful feeling flow over and spread through your entire body.

16. Keep a continuous feeling of moving forward into the light as it is drawn into you and you are drawn into it.

17. Your body should feel extremely comfortable. Remain perfectly still to maintain that blissful comfort.

18. There is a subtle nerve channel that runs from under the right eye, down the cheek, to the bottom of the jawbone, then along the lower jaw to its hinge, and back up behind the right ear. Turning your attention to this nadi will lead you from the light to the sound.

19. With a feeling of unconditional love and sense of joyful anticipation, invite the Inner Sacred Sound to arise.

20. Trust that the sound is already vibrating within you.

21. Allowing the sound to arise is something we intuitively and naturally know how to do. With unconditional love surrender your control over the sound.

22. Listen through the right ear for an internal sound. The sound may take many forms: a low rumble, a buzzing, a resonant sustained tone, a shimmering tinkle, or a high ringing. If you don't hear any of these right away, be patient and wait with a joyful anticipation for the sound to arise. Allow for the possibility that in time you will hear it.

23. If sound arises, hold it in your attention without trying to control it. Thank it with unconditional love for arising.

24. It is a very subtle sound. Whatever sound you hear, fix your attention on the subtlest part of it: the sound behind, above, within, or beyond the sound. Just by focusing on the subtlest part, it will increase in intensity and volume.

25. Follow the sound, co-absorb with it, letting it pour into you, filling you like water from a pitcher.

26. Having co-absorbed with both the sound and the light, realize you are not separate from them. You and the light are one. You and the sound are one. The light is the sound. The sound is the light. You and the light and the sound are all merged. Dissolve into them and them into you. You are all one.

27. Remain perfectly still in your body and mind.

33 ✸ The Basic Meditation with Simple Instructions

Focus on the sound and bliss will come from the attainment of Reality.

GHERANDA SAMHITA 7.10

1. Sit in siddhasana or on a blanket or pillow with pressure on your perineum.
2. Block your ears with earplugs.
3. Put your hands on your knees. Keep your spine straight.
4. Close your eyes.
5. Sit comfortably in complete stillness.
6. Rest in your heart, with unconditional love.
7. Look up between your eyebrows. Make this effortless, without strain.
8. Trust that the light is already shining within us. Surrender to it.
9. Quiet your mind.
10. Watch for flickering, clouds or rays of color, or lights.
11. If light arises, with unconditional love thank it.
12. Steadily concentrate on it until, over time, it becomes a single focused point.
13. Co-absorb with the light by moving it into the center of your head.
14. As you do so pull your eyes back in toward the center of your head.

15. Let the light spread over your head and around your body.

16. Continue moving forward into the light.

17. Remain perfectly still to maintain the feeling of blissful comfort.

18. Mentally trace the subtle nerve channel, from below the right eye to behind the right ear.

19. With unconditional love, invite the Inner Sacred Sound to arise.

20. With unconditional love, surrender your control over the sound.

21. Trust that the sound already *is* vibrating within you.

22. Listen for sound within your right ear.

23. If sound arises, thank it with unconditional love.

24. Listen for the subtlest part of the sound. It will get louder.

25. Pull the sound from your ear into yourself, filling your head and body.

26. Dissolve into the sound and the light as one.

27. Remain perfectly still in your body and mind.

PART SEVEN

Additive Practices

34 ✺ Six Additions

The highest of all absorptions is nada yoga, from which the highest form of samadhi will arise.

YOGA TARAVALI 2

Here are some additional elements that can be integrated into the Basic Practice to strengthen and deepen its overall effects.

TONGUE PLACEMENT

Place your tongue on the front of the roof of your mouth. The whole front of the tongue should be resting lightly across the ridge just at the root of the upper front teeth. It should be relaxed and without tension.

BANDHAS

Bandha means "to bind." These are physical locks done by contracting a specific musculature within the body.

There are primarily three bandhas: mula bandha, uddiyana bandha, and jalandhara bandha. Only the first two are used here. The third, jalandhara bandha, should be learned from a competent yoga teacher as a part of pranayama.

Mula Bandha

Mula Bandha means "root lock." It is the drawing up of the perineum by contracting the pubococcygeus (PC) muscle. The PC is the muscle that is engaged when Kegel exercises are done. It can be isolated during urination by contracting it to stop the flow. In mula bandha the PC muscle is held lightly in contraction. Mula bandha causes prana to rise from the perineum, passing in front of the spine to the top of the head.

You may notice a slight shift in your vision or a feeling of focus as you engage mula bandha. This is the energy moving upward.

Uddiyana Bandha

This bandha is a pulling in and up of the stomach muscles about three finger-widths below the navel. This is a light contraction. *Uddiyana* means "flying up." It causes the energy to rise and shift your consciousness.

My teacher, Pattabhi Jois, taught both mula bandha and uddiyana bandha as a part of the ashtanga yoga practice. He taught that "these are the anal and lower abdominal locks that seal in energy, give lightness, strength and health to the body, and help to build a strong internal fire."[1] They are also helpful in focusing attention in nada yoga.

MANTRA

Mantra can now be applied to the first part of the basic meditation. If you are distracted by your thoughts while looking between the brows, chant *So* on the inhale and *Ham* on the exhale. Other possible mantras to use are Om or a personal mantra. If you choose a mantra other than *So'ham,* repeat it both on the inhale and the exhale. This will help stem the tide of thoughts as you look at the light. Once you have co-absorbed with the light and begin listening for the nada, let go of repeating the mantra.

SECOND POINT OF FOCUS

Once you have co-absorbed with both the light and the sound, look straight ahead, *through* your eyelids, as if you are looking at a point far in the distance. You will experience the broadening of vision and feeling of relaxation that occurs when looking at a far-off mountain or across a great body of water. The sense of physical space surrounding you may expand into a vast openness, a distant horizon, an expansive pale white sky. Although you should maintain a sustained focus, actively looking, your eyes should be relaxed.

THE BREATH

On the inhale draw the energy up from the base of your spine to the top of your head. This is a twofold action. On the inhale, as the breath expands and pushes down on the diaphragm, this builds a light pressure in the lower abdomen. This pressure causes a slight pumping action of the energy at the base of the spine.

At the same time there is a pulling up of the energy from the top of the head as if you are creating a vacuum there that pulls the energy up the spine. This feels like pulling liquid up through a straw. As you inhale both things happen simultaneously. As you exhale you let the energy recede back down your spine.

GROUNDING

After meditation, we need to be fully awake and back in our bodies so we can safely interact with the world around us. If we are not fully present on the physical plane, we can lose track and injure ourselves. To come into full awareness, rub your head, neck, arms, torso, legs, and especially the bottoms of your feet. Focus on the feeling of your body as you do so.

In the next two chapters the meditation with additions will be presented in two forms: the first with full in-depth instructions, the second with simple one-line instructions. Again, as in chapters 32 and 33, the repetition and condensation of the instructions in chapters 35 and 36 are to encourage you to condense the instructions further in your self-practice. Chapter 37 reduces the practice to five simple sentences.

35 ✳ Meditation with Additions, Full Instructions

Don't have a single thought. Let all of them go, both thoughts of the external and the internal.

HATHA YOGA PRADIPIKA 4.57

Here is the meditation with the additive practices integrated in, with instructions for each step.

1. Take a couple of deep slow breaths, with equal inhale and exhale. Then let your breathing settle into a relaxed, easy flow.

2. Sit comfortably with your body in symmetry. Let the right side of your body (hands/arms, feet/legs) be in the same position as the left side. If you can sit with your legs crossed with one of your heels pressing up into your perineum, that is ideal. If not, sit on a rolled up blanket or pillow with your legs on both sides so that there is pressure on your perineum. Block the sound entering your ears with earplugs. You can use your fingers instead, although this will cause a sound of its own, which may be distracting.

3. Put your hands on your knees. This will prevent you from slumping. Keep your spine straight. (If your fingers are in your ears, sit with your feet flat on the ground and your knees up. Put your elbows on your knees.)

4. Rest your tongue on the front of the roof of your mouth with the tip resting lightly on the ridge just above the roots of the upper teeth.

5. Close your eyes.

6. Lightly engage mula bandha, by contracting the PC muscle, and uddiyana bandha, by pulling the belly in and the navel up. This will help the energy move up from the perineum, passing in front of the spine, all the way to the top of the head.

7. Try to find a position of comfort so you don't have to move. You want to be able to sit in perfect stillness in order for yoga nidra to arise.

8. Recall a past experience of unconditional love. Fill your heart with that feeling. Repose in the center of your heart, suffused with that unconditional love.

9. With your eyes still closed look up between your eyebrows. Your gaze is inward, but your focus is as if you were looking outward into the distance. Although you are actively looking/watching, try to make this effortless, without strain.

10. With a feeling of unconditional love and sense of joyful anticipation, invite the Divine Light to arise.

11. Allowing the light to arise is something we intuitively and naturally know how to do. The light is already shining within us. With unconditional love surrender your control over it.

12. Quiet your mind. Let go of all thinking. If thoughts come up, let them pass like a cloud in the sky. Then bring your focus back to looking/watching between your eyebrows.

13. If you continue to be distracted by your thoughts, chant *So* on the inhale and *Ham* on the exhale, or Om, or a personal mantra. If you would rather use a word in English that is meaningful, *One* or *Love* will work nicely. Repeat it both on the inhale and the exhale.

14. At first you may see only darkness. Eventually you will begin to see flickering, clouds, rays of color, or lights. These are not imagined. They are an internal perception.

15. If light arises, hold it in your attention without trying to control it. Thank it with unconditional love for arising.

16. With continuous unbroken concentration, over time, the lights will eventually become a single focused point of light. It may be a very small, intense dot or fleck of light, an iridescent blue or indigo "pearl" surrounded by a corona, a bright burning ball of white light, a shimmering star, or other concentrations of brilliant radiance.

17. Realize that you are not separate from the light. Embrace that "You are that." Co-absorb with the light by moving it into the center of your head.

18. At the same time draw your eyes back in toward the center of your head, pulling the light with them.

19. Draw the light into and around you. As you dissolve into it and it into you, blissfully feel it surrounding and covering your head. Let that blissful feeling flow over and spread through your entire body.

20. Keep a continuous feeling of moving forward into the light as it is drawn into you and you are drawn into it.

21. Your body should feel extremely comfortable. Remain perfectly still to maintain that blissful comfort.

22. Now that your attention has steadied, let go of any mantra you might be using. This clears the way for listening for the internal sound. The light leads the way to the sound.

23. There is a subtle nerve channel that runs from under the right eye, down the cheek to the bottom of the jawbone, along the lower jaw to its hinge, and back up behind the right ear. Turning your attention to this nadi will lead you from the light to the sound.

24. With a feeling of unconditional love and joyful anticipation, invite the Sacred Sound to arise.

25. Allowing the sound to arise is something we intuitively and naturally know how to do. The sound is already vibrating within us. With unconditional love, surrender your control over it.

26. Listen through the right ear for an internal sound. The sound may take many forms: a low rumble, a buzzing, a resonant sustained tone, a shimmering tinkle, or a high ringing. If you don't hear any of these right away, be patient and wait with a joyful anticipation for the sound to arise. Allow for the possibility that in time you will hear it.

27. If sound arises, hold it in your attention without trying to control it. Thank it with unconditional love for arising.

28. It is a very subtle sound. Whatever sound you hear fix your attention on the subtlest part of it: the sound behind, above, within, or beyond the sound. Just by focusing on it, it will increase in intensity and volume.

29. Follow the sound, co-absorb with it, letting it pour into you, filling you like water from a pitcher.

30. Having co-absorbed with both the sound and the light, realize you are not separate from them. You and the light are one. You and the sound are one. The light is the sound. The sound is the light. You and the light and the sound are all merged. Dissolve into them and them into you. You are all one.

31. Look straight ahead, "through" your eyelids, as if you are looking at a point far in the distance. You may experience a vast openness, a distant horizon, an expansive pale white sky.

32. On the inhale draw the breath/energy up from the perineum, up the spine, all the way to the top of the head. On the exhale let it release back down.

33. Dissolve the light, sound, breath/prana, and your mind all into one.

34. Remain perfectly still in your body and mind.

35. When you are finished rub your head, arms, torso, legs, and especially the bottoms of your feet.

36 ✸ Meditation with Additions, Simple Instructions

The entire universe is just a projection of the mind. The play of our thoughts is just a projection of mind.

HATHA YOGA PRADIPIKA 4.58

1. Take a few deep breaths.
2. Sit in siddhasana or on a blanket or pillow with pressure on your perineum.
3. Block the sound entering your ears with earplugs.
4. Put your hands on your knees. Keep your spine straight.
5. Place your tongue on the front of the roof of your mouth.
6. Close your eyes.
7. Lightly engage mula bandha and uddiyana bandha.
8. Sit comfortably in complete stillness.
9. Rest in your heart, with unconditional love.
10. Look up between your eyebrows. Make this effortless, without strain.
11. With unconditional love ask the Divine Light to arise.
12. Trust that we know how to let the light shining within us arise. Surrender to it.
13. Quiet your mind.
14. Repeat a mantra if it is helpful.

15. Watch for flickering lights, clouds or rays of light, or colors.

16. If light arises, thank it with unconditional love.

17. Steadily concentrate on it until, over time, it becomes a single focused point.

18. Co-absorb with the light by moving it into the center of your head.

19. As you do so, pull your eyes back in toward the center of your head.

20. Let the light spread over your head and around your body.

21. Continuously move forward into the light.

22. Remain perfectly still to maintain the feeling of blissful comfort.

23. Let go of the mantra if you are using one.

24. Follow the subtle nerve channel from just below the right eye to the right ear.

25. With unconditional love ask the Internal Sacred Sound to arise.

26. Trust that you know how to let the sound vibrating within you arise. Surrender to it.

27. Listen for sound within your right ear.

28. If sound arises, thank it with unconditional love.

29. Listen for the subtlest part of the sound. It will get louder.

30. Let the sound pour into your head and body.

31. Dissolve into the sound and light as one.

32. Look straight ahead "through" your eyelids at a point far in the distance.

33. On the inhale draw the breath/energy up your spine. On the exhale release it.

34. Dissolve the light, sound, breath/prana, and your mind all into one.

35. Remain perfectly still in your body and mind.

36. When finished rub your head, arms, body, legs, and bottoms of your feet.

37. Carry this new way of seeing/hearing into your daily life.

37 ❀ Meditation in Its Simplest Form

Empty inside, empty outside, empty like a pot in air. Full inside, full outside, full like a pot in the ocean.

HATHA YOGA PRADIPIKA 4.56

When you have gained some mastery of each of the components of the meditation, you will only need to remember these basic steps to recall all the previously learned information.

1. Sit comfortably in complete stillness.
2. Close your ears and eyes.
3. Rest in your heart with unconditional love.
4. Look up between your eyebrows.
5. Listen for sound within your right ear.

The final step is carrying this new way of seeing and hearing over into your daily life. The goal is to keep your eyes and ears open, to access feelings of unconditional love, concentration, and bliss, and to co-absorb with the universe and the people in it.

PART EIGHT

Supportive and Ancillary Practices

38 ✳ Asana

Perfection in asana is attained by letting go of effort and meditating on Reality.

YOGA SUTRAS 2.47

A practitioner of ashtanga yoga is doing his practice. As he glides through movements and comes to focused stillness in held postures, everything is measured by the breath. Standing up straight with his feet together (fig. 1), he inhales as he raises his arms overhead, brings his hands together, and looks up at his thumbs (fig. 2). On the exhale, he bends at the waist, his palms coming down to the ground next to the outside of his feet (fig. 3). Inhaling, he looks up and straightens his back (fig. 4). Still looking forward, he exhales, jumping back by straighten-

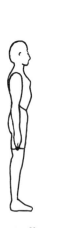 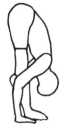 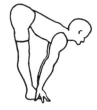

1. *Still* 2. *Inhale* 3. *Exhale* 4. *Inhale*

ing his legs, his feet shooting back behind where he had been standing. He lands parallel to the floor in a pushup position (fig. 5). Inhaling, he moves his chest forward between his arms, arching his back (fig. 6). Exhaling, he straightens his arms and bends at the waist, his body forming an inverted V (fig. 7). He holds this posture for five full inhales and exhales.

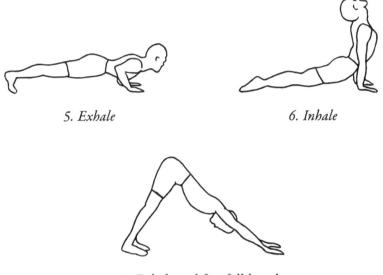

5. *Exhale*   6. *Inhale*

7. *Exhale and five full breaths*

Inhaling, he looks up and jumps his feet forward between his hands (fig. 8). Exhaling, he bends at the waist (fig. 9). Inhaling, he straightens up, raises his arms, brings his hands together overhead, and looks

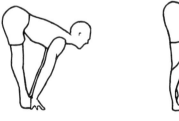

8. *Inhale*   9. *Exhale*

up (fig. 10). Exhaling, his arms come to his side. He is back where he started (fig. 11).

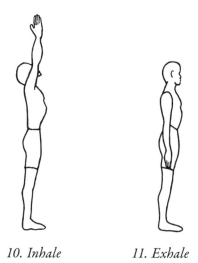

10. Inhale   *11. Exhale*

His breath drives his movements. We can hear this as well as see it. Although his mouth is closed, his breath is audible. It sounds like a distant ocean in his throat: the exhale, the sound of the wave breaking and rushing up onto the beach; the inhale, the sound of the water, drawn by gravity, pulling back to become part of the next wave. This cycle repeats again and again. This is *ujjayi* breath.

As he comes into a pose, he settles into holding it in stillness, all the while continuing his ujjayi breath. In addition he fixes his gaze on a specific point, whether it is at the tip of his nose, on his hand, on his navel, between his eyebrows, or any of the total of nine *drishti,* points of visual focus. Each posture has a specific drishti.

Ashtanga is one of myriad styles and types of yoga asana practiced around the world. It is wonderful that there are so many lineages to choose from in the practice of asana. We all learn in different ways. The specifics of asana practice are far too broad a subject to cover here in any depth. I recommend that you find a teacher and style of yoga asana that engages you physically, mentally, and spiritually.

YOGA ASANA TEACHERS

Yoga asana practice is an ancient method for the realization of the Self. Its knowledge and wisdom have evolved by being passed down and refined, from teacher to student, over many millennia.

Find a qualified teacher from an established lineage that reaches back through time. In other words, find out who your teacher's teacher's teacher was. Find a teacher whom you feel you can trust, someone with a depth of knowledge of the material they are teaching and the wisdom attained through life experience applied to that knowledge, someone whose touch supports and facilitates the opening of your body and mind, someone who has the ability to teach to each student's individual needs and way of learning. The way you learn should also determine the style of asana you choose.

YOGA ASANA STYLES

Asana should challenge you over time, with regular practice, to slowly open your joints, muscles, and their connections to your skeletal system. Choose a style that helps you squeeze and pump your internal organs, cleansing toxins by increasing circulation and promoting the flow of prana. Ideally it should also build strength, muscle mass, and bone density. As well as opening the body and bringing about physical change, it should make positive changes in the way you think, relate to others, and see the world around you.

VINYASA

A *vinyasa* is a movement linked to the breath. Many styles of yoga asana include vinyasa. We can trace the roots of the lineage that fostered vinyasa back to a cave in the mountains of Tibet. It was there that T. Krishnamacharya studied with Ramamohana Brahmachari for more than seven years. Krishnamacharya went on to teach Sri K. Pattabhi

Jois and T. K. V. Desikachar. Vinyasa is a fundamental part both of their teachings of asana practice.

The description at the beginning of this chapter of the ashtanga yogi doing his practice includes several vinyasa. A vinyasa is often done between held postures. By moving with breath after holding a posture, vinyasa brings the body back to neutral. It wipes the slate clean in preparation for the next posture.

In *surya namaskara* (sun salutes) we do a series of several vinyasas, which include moving through *urdhva mukha svanasana* (upward facing dog, fig. 6) with an inhale, to *adho mukha svanasana* (downward facing dog, fig. 7) with an exhale. These movements bring us through positions in which our head is above our body and then positions in which our head is lower than most of our body.

We are repeatedly infusing our brain with freshly oxygenated blood by doing these movements with deep relaxed breathing. At the same time we are increasing the circulation of cerebrospinal fluid that washes away the waste bi-products of the brain and spine and passes them back out through the blood-brain barrier for excretion. These two processes physically nourish and clear the brain, preparing the mind to focus. After six or seven surya namaskaras our mind starts to come to a clarity it did not have before doing them.

By the repetition of vinyasa we also strengthen the cerebral blood vessels that control blood flow to the brain. In any inversion blood rushes to the head. The blood vessels contract to stop too much blood from rushing to the brain and causing damage. The repetition of going in and out of inversion as we do in vinyasa causes a repetition of the contraction and dilation of these blood vessels. The immediate effect of this action is to aid circulation. Over time the repeated contraction and dilation strengthens the contractive capability of these vessels. This makes them more responsive to surges in blood pressure, greatly reducing our susceptibility to stroke.

Vinyasa encourages the flow of both our circulatory and lymphatic systems, brings our body back to neutral, and detoxifies both the brain and body. Vinyasa prepares the mind to focus and the body to sit in asana in stillness.

WHY DO WE PRACTICE ASANA?

There are the obvious reasons for practice: It makes us feel better physically, lighter, more flexible, stronger. It makes us look better. A diligent daily practice will no doubt give us a firm, finely toned body. There are, however, some important qualities of asana that can enhance, not only our lives, but support our nada yoga meditation practice.

Contemporary psychology equates our emotional state with our posture. If we are feeling "down," our shoulders and spine are often slumped, our head is tilted forward, our eyes are cast downward. When we are feeling "up," our shoulders and spine are straight, our face is slightly lifted, and our eyes have a higher focus.

By changing our physical posture we can change our psychological state. If we are feeling down, simply by straightening our shoulders and spine, lifting our head, and looking up we can lift our mood. The body sends the message to the brain: *I'm in my feeling good position.* The brain responds by starting to feel good.

If physiology affects our mood, then imagine the power of realigning and opening the body in new ways while the breath is relaxed and the mind is focused. When we put our foot behind our head for the first time and our ankle touches the back of our neck, we experience a physical sensation we have never had before. By touching two parts of our body together that have never made physical contact, we are connecting nerve endings that have never touched. These nerves fire simultaneously and cause synapses in the brain to also fire simultaneously. This forms a new neural pathway.

If simply changing our physiology changes our mood, then new postures and physical connections that create new neural pathways make possible new ways of thinking and being.

Many yoga teachers will tell you that the reason you do asana is so that you can sit in meditation. One might think that means that when you have finished your asana practice you will be relaxed enough and your body will be open enough to sit for a few minutes. Although that is true, there are other long-term effects of asana practice that are helpful in meditation. Through asana we challenge ourselves to open our body and our mind. We cultivate the ability to sit in absolute stillness, the ability to focus our mind, the ability to cast off old patterns and ways of being and move toward a higher consciousness. Stillness, focus, and change are ways asana aids us in finding the bliss of nada yoga meditation and the path toward the larger, lofty goal of enlightenment.

STILLNESS

When we do asana regularly, over a long period of time, we are training our body to sit in complete stillness. This is sometimes in spite of slight discomfort. Holding a posture for an extended period of time is challenging. As the body opens and we hold or deepen a pose, that feeling of slight discomfort becomes familiar and sometimes disappears altogether. We may then attempt a more difficult variation of that pose to start the process all over again. As our body opens it begins to quiet down and settle, letting go of our need to fidget and squirm. As the body comes to complete stillness, there is a parallel quieting of the mind.

FOCUS

The mind loves to play. In a yoga asana class it can sometimes run freely from thought to thought, in judgment or self-criticism: *"Oh, look at them, they can't do this pose at all . . . Oh, look at them, they are amazing . . . I'll never be able to do this pose . . . Oh, look at me, I can really do this next pose. . . ."* and on and on. But if we are trying to do a balance pose and internal dialogue starts, and we lose track of our body, our breath, and our point of focus, we won't be able to hold the balance.

In ashtanga yoga we have *tristhana,* three points of attention: posture, breath, and a point of visual focus. These teach the mind to stay focused in the present moment. We learn to avoid distractions, whether they are in our external world or in our inner dialogue. Other forms of yoga have similar tools to cultivate focus.

We can see in this process the steps of 1) turning our senses inward away from distraction (*pratyahara*), 2) repeatedly returning our mind to concentration on the posture (*dharana*), and 3) settling into a continuous state of connection with the pose (*dhyana*).

Regular and sustained practice over a long period of time will bring an ease and immediacy to the focusing of the mind.

ENLIGHTENMENT

Self-realization, illumination, or awakening to Reality all seem distant and unattainable. For some, it happens in the flash of a moment. More often than not, it is a long path that is a continuum rather than an instantaneous change.

Although it is a realm reached by very few, we still work toward that state, hopefully both on the mat and in our daily lives. What is it that we are doing in asana practice that helps us move toward that goal? How does asana bring about these changes?

Through events and relationships in our lives we sometimes experience trauma and injury to our bodies and our psyche. These events cause both emotional and physical reactions in the body.

The emotional reactions can be reflected in brain chemistry, hormones, and other biochemical balancing processes. At the same time the physical reaction can cause contraction, misalignment, or desensitization of parts of our body.

The impact on both emotions and the body happens at the same time; they are intertwined. We store the emotional experiences in both our bodies and our brains. These experiences shape how we will react to the people and world around us in the future. Through repetition of these reactions, they become habitual patterns.

If every time we speak someone yells "Be quiet!" we begin to prevent ourselves from speaking. Both the stress of the expectation of getting yelled at and the internal conflict of wanting to speak and stopping ourselves set off reactions in our brain and body.

In the brain there is a stress response that causes a biochemical spike. To protect ourselves from being yelled at again, our brain goes into the hyper-vigilance of the "fight or flight" response. Our awareness sharpens to the point that it makes us highly reactive.

To prevent ourselves from speaking we might clench our jaw every time we want to speak. This constant contraction of the jaw muscles can affect the muscles in the neck and upper back. If this goes on for a long time, all of these muscles may go into a constant state of tightness or contraction.

The physical reaction and emotional reaction are simultaneous. The body captures both the contraction of the muscle and the biochemical spike in the brain, storing a kind of emotional profile of each trauma. Both reactions are linked as a single event.

As we do asana the body stretches and opens. Those places in contraction resist the opening. This causes discomfort. In many cases the area in contraction has been desensitized and numbed. Our ability to feel it is outside of our usual conscious awareness.

As we sit in asana, the mild discomfort draws our attention to the contracted, neglected area. By doing so we light up the synapses in our brain at the site of the stored trauma. Just as the trauma in the body and the brain are intertwined, the opening in the body and the release in the mind also happen simultaneously.

If we continue to stretch and open the affected area with regular committed practice, we release some of the biochemical profile of our past emotional experiences. As they are released we are freed from the ingrained habitual patterns and reactivity that have built up over time as a result of physical and emotional trauma.

In yoga philosophy these constrictions can be seen in a similar, parallel model. The nadis are a vast network of 72,000 nerve channels that run throughout our entire body. They regulate and channel our energy, our prana. The three most important nadis are the *ida* (moon), *pingala* (sun), and *sushumna* (center).

All three start at the *muladhara* chakra at the base of the spine. The sushumna nadi runs straight up in front of the spine to the *sahasrara* chakra at the crown of the head. The ida and pingala nadis run alongside the sushumna, simultaneously crossing it at five points. These crossing points are where the other five chakras lie.

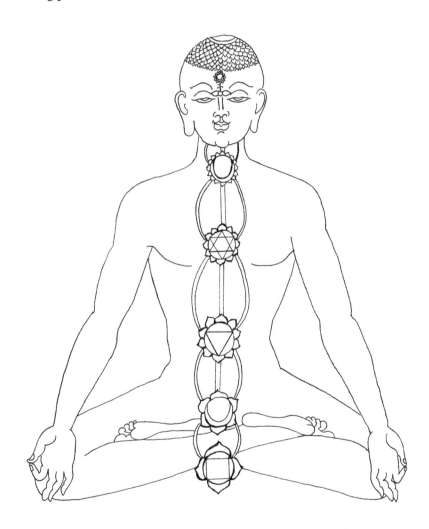

Chakras

The ida nadi and pingala nadi meet at the *ajna* chakra between the eyebrows. From there they descend down the left nostril (ida) and right nostril (pingala) where they end.

In yogic philosophy one becomes enlightened when prana from the ida and pingala nadis enter the sushumna nadi and ascends, without obstruction, to the crown chakra.

The nadis and chakras are a latticework within the brain, which is projected as a kind of virtual overlay within the body. Chakras, although not physical structures, each have a correlation to a point on the sushumna, which lies along the body's center line. There is a predominate emotional attribute at each of the intersections at the chakras. If there is trauma to an emotional attribute, the correlating chakra becomes constricted or blocked. This prevents prana from entering and rising to the crown chakra and the attainment of enlightenment.

These constrictions and blockages are the effect of negative proclivities and tendencies known as *samskaras*. Samskaras are the seeds of our past actions, karma. They accrue and blossom, holding us in an unending cycle of habitual patterns.

By opening the body through the practice of asana, we start to burn the seeds of samskaras so they cannot blossom. This in turn loosens the constrictions of the chakras. This enables the prana to begin to enter and rise up the sushumna.

This opening, release, and loosening of impediments through asana supports, expedites, and deepens the practice of nada yoga. Although it may take many small steps, asana can, together with meditation, help us begin the long journey toward enlightenment.

It is in our nature to avoid discomfort. Asana forces us to confront our discomfort, move through it, and learn from it. By doing so we attain strength and range of motion in both our body and our mind. Yoga asana practice gives us the tools we need to sit in comfort with our discomfort: stillness, focus, and motivation to bring ourselves to a state of higher consciousness.

39 ✸ Pranayama

Pranayama lifts the veil of ignorance from the Inner Light.
YOGA SUTRAS 2.52

PRANAYAMA

The very first thing we do when we are born on this planet is take a nice big inhale. The last thing we do is gently exhale. The average person breathes around 21,600 times a day. Even with a conservative life span of seventy years, that's approximately 551,880,000 breaths. Most of them are well outside our conscious awareness unless we purposefully focus on the breath.

If we had to think about our breath to keep it going, we either wouldn't be able to do anything else or we wouldn't survive very long. What a miraculous thing it is that, without even thinking about it, we continue to inhale and take oxygen into our lungs and body and exhale and put out carbon dioxide and thus stay alive.

As children our breathing is regulated by how physically active we are and what emotions we are feeling. If a child is upset and crying, their breathing completely changes from its normal cycle. Even after they have stopped crying, their diaphragm keeps moving. They still have a hitch in their breath as their diaphragm contracts in spasm.

Our breathing patterns become more set as we become adults. We learn to "control" the outward expression of our emotions. When our emotions are particularly strong, our bodies don't always comply. If we

135

are upset or angry, our breathing may become constricted as we try to control our feelings. As a result our voice may become shaky or shrill.

If we lead a physically inactive life, we may use less of our lungs to breathe. If we sit in a chair much of the day, we may only use the top one-third or even one-quarter of our lungs.

If we have stress in our lives, we may have a continuous "fight or flight" response, causing our breathing to become shallow and rapid much of the time.

If we are calm and relaxed, our breathing becomes slow, soft, and regular.

Strong feeling or emotions will alter our breathing, making it quick and ragged.

❀ Breath Awareness Meditation

1. As you travel through your day check your breathing by resting your hand on your chest or belly.
2. Notice how different positions you are in affect your breathing.
3. Notice how different ways of moving affect your breathing.
4. Notice how different thoughts or feelings affect your breathing.
5. Notice when your breathing is fast.
6. Notice when your breathing is slow.
7. Notice when your breathing is deep.
8. Notice when your breathing is shallow.
9. Notice when your breathing is smooth and regular.
10. Notice when your breathing is irregular or ragged.
11. Notice when you hold your breath.

PRANAYAMA PRACTICE

Ancient yogis understood that if we control the breath, we control our state of mind. If we change our breathing patterns, we change our mental and emotional state.

Prana is a Sanskrit word meaning breath, vital energy, life force.

Yama means to restrain or control. Pranayama is the fourth limb of yoga. T. K. V. Desikachar defines it as "the conscious, deliberate regulation of the breath replacing unconscious patterns of breathing."[1]

There are many kinds of pranayama, or breath control, that have different effects on the body and mind. Its practice purifies the nervous system and can energize, relax, and balance the body. If you are interested in practicing pranayama, I strongly suggest that you find an experienced yoga teacher to work with you individually. As an introduction here are two beginning forms.

UJJAYI BREATH

Ujjayi breathing is a pranayama in which we add sound to the inhale and exhale. We do so to use both our kinesthetic sense and our sense of hearing to keep our breath in our conscious awareness. This pranayama was previously mentioned as a part of ashtanga yoga practice and described as sounding like ocean waves breaking and receding on a beach.

❊ *Ujjayi Pranayama*

1. Sit comfortably with your back straight and your body in left-right symmetry.
2. Hold your palm 4 to 6 inches in front of your mouth, as if it were a pane of glass.
3. As you exhale slightly constrict the bottom of your throat, making a *haaaaa* sound as if fogging up the glass with the moisture from your breath.
4. As you inhale make the same sound.
5. Make this sound for the entire inhale and exhale.
6. Breathe through your nose with your mouth closed with this sound.
7. Extend your inhale by slowly counting to five.
8. As you exhale slowly count to five.
9. Make your inhale and exhale smooth and of equal length and intensity.
10. Inhale and then exhale five times in this way.

✺ *Alternate Nostril Pranayama*

This pranayama has a calming effect, slowing the breath and heart rate. It is a good treatment for insomnia.

1. Hold up your right-hand palm facing you with your first two fingers bent and your thumb, ring finger, and little finger straight (fig. 1).

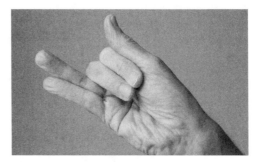

1. Finger Position

2. Close your mouth.
3. Lightly press your ring finger on the left side of your nose, closing your left nostril (fig. 2).

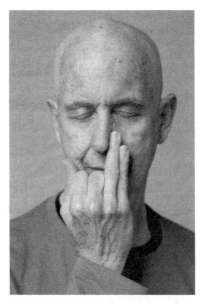

2. Close left nostril

4. Inhale through your right nostril for a slow count of five.

5. Release your ring finger from your left nostril.

6. Lightly press your thumb on the right side of your nose, closing your right nostril (fig. 3).

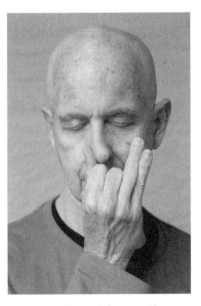

3. Close right nostril

7. Exhale through your left nostril for a slow count of five.

8. With your thumb still holding the right nostril shut, inhale through the left nostril for a slow count of five.

9. Release your thumb from your right nostril.

10. Again, press your ring finger on the left side of your nose, closing your left nostril. Exhale through your right nostril for a slow count of five.

11. The transition between the inhale and exhale should be smooth and without pause.

12. One round is: inhale right, exhale left, inhale left, exhale right.

13. Do three complete rounds.

40 ✵ The Eight Limbs

*Through the practice of the Eight Limbs of Yoga, we are
purified, and the Light of Wisdom shows us the difference
between illusion and Reality.*

YOGA SUTRAS 2.28

Within Patanjali's teaching on the precepts for the practice of yoga,
the *Yoga Sutras* are the Eight Limbs of Yoga. Pattabhi Jois taught that
we begin the eight limbs with the third limb, asana practice. We then
progress from there. His belief was, the deeper we became involved
with our asana practice, the more we would naturally want to live
our life according to the teachings of the first two limbs, *yamas* and
niyamas.

So far we have looked at the third limb, asana, and a fourth limb,
pranayama. Here are all eight limbs in the order they are presented in
the *Yoga Sutras*. Their totality encourages the self-discovery that takes
place within our nada meditation. They also show us how to carry that
practice back into the world around us.

I. YAMAS (ABSTINENCES)

The yamas are five instructions on moral attitudes and actions in relationship to the world around us. They are a code of conduct for how
to treat others. They are: *ahimsa* (non-harming in thought, word, and
action), *satya* (truthfulness, honesty, and sincerity), *asteya* (non-stealing),

140

brahmacharya (celibacy or control of our sexual energy), and *aparigraha* (non-greed).

2. NIYAMAS (OBSERVANCES)

The niyamas are five instructions on moral attitudes and actions in relationship to ourselves. They are a code of conduct for how we are within our own being. They are: *saucha* (purity, cleanliness), *samtosa* (contentment), *tapas* ("to burn" impurities through vigorous physical or mental practice), *svadhyaya* (study of self and spiritual texts), and *isvarapranidhanani* (devotion to the Divine).

3. ASANA (STILL AND COMFORTABLE PHYSICAL POSTURE)

Asana literally means "seat." It applies to many different physical postures taken with intention. Asana was explored in greater depth in chapter 38.

4. PRANAYAMA (BREATH CONTROL, OR REGULATION)

There are many forms of pranayama that lengthen, strengthen, or retain the breath to alter one's physical and mental state. Pranayama was explored in greater depth in chapter 39.

5. PRATYAHARA (WITHDRAWAL FROM THE ORGANS OF THE SENSES)

If, in spite of external sights, sounds, and tactile sensation, we can focus the pathways of our vision, hearing, and kinesthetic sense on the internal perceptions of the inner emanating light, the Inner Sacred Sound, and the feelings of internal vibration and bliss, this is pratyahara.

6. DHARANA (CONCENTRATION)

We sometimes speak of someone's power of concentration. It is an observation about a person's ability to stay focused on what they are doing no matter what is going on around them. By developing pratyahara we turn our senses inward, away from the distractions in the world around us.

Once we have turned our gaze, our listening, and our kinesthetic sense inward, we may then be distracted by what dominates our internal world: our thought processes, our monkey mind jumping from thought to thought. Developing our powers of concentration in our internal world is a skill that is developed over time with practice. It is the ability to keep our attention returning to one "object." This cultivation of concentration is the starting place for the next step, dhyana.

7. DHYANA (MEDITATION)

Meditation is holding concentration without the intrusion of other thoughts. It is when the bond of your focus on the "object" is so strong that nothing can distract you. When this unbroken connection is established, it allows for the eighth limb, *samadhi*, to occur.

8. SAMADHI (COMPLETE CO-ABSORPTION WITH UNIVERSAL CONSCIOUSNESS)

When the consciousness of the meditator, the stable concentration, and the "object" of concentration become integrated so they are fused and indistinguishable, this is samadhi.

Within the texts of both the *Hatha Yoga Pradipika* and the *Yoga Sutras,* the words "dissolve" and "absorption" occur often. They are variations on the translation of samadhi. There are between two and eight levels of samadhi, depending on which teaching you follow. Initially we hope to attain the first and most basic level of samadhi as a result of our meditation.

SAMYAMA

In the *Yoga Sutras* the last three limbs are garlanded together into *samyama*. There is a line, or thread, which starts with turning our senses inward (pratyahara). The line runs through, focusing our attention (dharana). When our attention becomes unbroken, we enter meditation (dhyana). Finally, when the meditator, the meditation, and the "object" being meditated upon become one, each indistinguishable from the other, we have the cohesion of samadhi. When the last three: dharana, dhyana, and samadhi, come together in succession, it is called samyama.

41 ✸ The Chakras

When the yogi meditates on the crown chakra, a brilliant light as bright as lightning is seen.

SHIVA SAMHITA 5.62

The chakras are energy centers within the body along the center channel, the sushumna, which runs up in front of the spine. The chakras are where the other two main nadis, or nerve channels, the ida and pingala, intersect with the sushumna nadi. Although the chakras aren't a physical organ or anatomical structure, there is a specific correlation between each of the chakras and a location along the body's center line. (See the illustration on page 133.)

Down through the millennia, using meditation, yogis have codified the attributes of each chakra. As well as location, there is also a shape, color, sound, and element intrinsic to each of the chakras.

Specific types of habitual patterns, in different parts of our lives, are related to different chakras. Meditating on each chakra; feeling its location; visualizing its projected shape, emanating color, and related element; and repeating its seed sound mantra brings awareness of constriction, blockages, or impurities that may exist.

Awareness of these impediments begins the process of loosening, opening, and purifying the chakras, freeing us of our habitual patterns. This will promote the flow of prana into and up the sushumna.

FIRST CHAKRA

Sanskrit name: Muladhara chakra
English name: Root, base
Location: Perineum
Shape: Square
Emanating color: Red
Element: Earth
Sound: Lahm
Aspect: Survival

SECOND CHAKRA

Sanskrit name: Svadhishthana chakra
English name: Home or dwelling place
Location: Three finger-widths below the navel
Shape: Crescent moon
Emanating color: Orange
Element: Water
Sound: Vahm
Aspect: Desire, sexuality

THIRD CHAKRA

Sanskrit name: Manipura chakra
English name: City of jewels
Location: Solar plexus
Shape: Triangle
Emanating color: Yellow
Element: Fire
Sound: Rahm
Aspect: Power

FOURTH CHAKRA

Sanskrit name: Anahata chakra
English name: The unstruck, sustained
Location: Center of the chest
Shape: Six-pointed star
Emanating color: Green
Element: Air
Sound: Yahm
Aspect: Unconditional love

FIFTH CHAKRA

Sanskrit name: Vishuddha chakra
English name: Pure
Location: Base of the throat
Shape: Circle
Emanating color: Blue
Element: Akasha (space)
Sound: Hahm
Aspect: Expression, communication

SIXTH CHAKRA

Sanskrit name: Ajna chakra
English name: To command, will, or summon
Location: Between the eyebrows
Shape: A single point
Emanating color: Violet, indigo
Element: All five elements in their purest form
Sound: Om, or the Inner Sacred Sound
Aspect: Insight, the gate to realization

SEVENTH CHAKRA

Sanskrit name: Sahasrara chakra
English name: Thousand-petaled lotus
Location: Crown of the head
Shape: Infinite space
Emanating color: White light
Element: Infinite time
Sound: Para (beyond sound)
Aspect: Transcendence, Universal Consciousness

✳ *Chakra Meditation*

1. Come into your meditative seat.
2. Visualize a box of red earth at the base of your spine over the perineum. Internally hear the sound *lahm.*
3. Visualize an orange crescent moon over water in front of your spine three finger-widths below your navel. Internally hear the sound *vahm.*
4. Visualize a yellow pyramid in flames in front of your spine at the solar plexus. Internally hear the sound *rahm.*
5. Visualize a green six-pointed star in front of your spine at the center of your chest. Internally hear the sound *yahm.*
6. Visualize a blue sphere at the base of your throat. Internally hear the sound *hahm.*
7. Visualize a single violet, indigo point between your eyebrows. Internally hear the sound *Om.*
8. Imagine the top of your head is covered by a lotus flower with a thousand petals. Visualize each of the petal tips rising off your head, forming a blossom from which a brilliant pure white light is emanating into infinite space.

✳ *Chakra Sound Meditation*

1. Come into your meditative seat.
2. Concentrate on the crown chakra.

3. Sing a long tone in the upper midrange of your voice.

4. Physically and energetically focus the tone on the crown of your head.

5. Use the mouth, the tongue, the throat, the bronchia, and the spine to physically direct the sound.

6. Try different tones until you find one that increases the amount of vibration.

7. Repeat steps 3 through 6 for each of the other six chakras, lowering the tones as you move downward to the base of the spine.

BEYOND THE SEVEN CHAKRAS

In Gorakshanath's writings there are nine chakras. As well as the two additional chakras, the placement and names of some of the other seven chakras are different from those listed above.

The second chakra, svadhishthana, is located at the genitals instead of just below the navel. The third chakra, manipura, is located at the navel instead of the solar plexus. The fourth and fifth chakras are the same as listed above.

Gorakshanath adds a sixth chakra at the root of the soft palate. He calls it the talu chakra. Because of the addition of the talu chakra, the ajna chakra then becomes the seventh chakra. He calls it the *bhru* or eyebrow chakra.

In Gorakshanath's system the eighth chakra is the nirvana chakra. This replaces the lotus skullcap of the sahasrara chakra with a single point. The nirvana chakra is at the top of the sushumna nadi within the *brahmarandha* or Brahmic opening, what we today call the fontanel. The additional ninth chakra is the akasha chakra, the chakra of empty radiant space. It is at the very top of the head, directly above the eighth chakra.

Gorakshanath places great importance on the talu chakra, calling it the tenth door. The other nine doors are the eyes, ears, nostrils, mouth, genitals, and anus. These other doors open to the world with prana flowing in and out. On the other hand, when the prana moves upward through the tenth door of the talu chakra, it moves through the chakras above it to re-unite us with Universal Consciousness.

42 ✳ Neti

Neti purifies the head, gives divine sight, and destroys disease above the shoulders.

HATHA YOGA PRADIPIKA 2.30

Use of the neti pot is a *kriya,* an action of purification, a form of internal cleansing of the body.

Although not necessary for everyone, using a neti pot daily is helpful in balancing the ida and pingala channels, clearing the nasal passages for pranayama, and the treatment of congestion due to sinus problems or allergies.

A neti pot can be bought at most natural food stores. It is a small spouted pot that looks like a little Aladdin's lamp. It holds about a cup of water.

✳ *Neti Pot Practice*

1. Add I teaspoon of non-iodine sea salt to a quart (4 cups) of distilled or spring water.
2. Heat to a little bit warmer than lukewarm.
3. Fill the neti pot.
4. Stand with your face tipped forward over a sink.
5. Breathe through your mouth.
6. Insert the spout of the pot into the left nostril so that it seals.
7. Raise the handle of the pot so the water pours into your left nostril.
8. Tip your head slightly to the right so that the water flows up through your left nasal passage and pours out your right nostril.

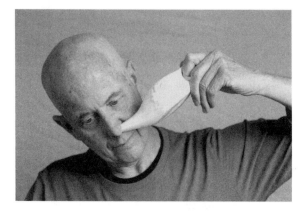

Neti pot position

9. Once the pot has emptied, refill it and insert the spout into your right nostril, letting the water flow out your left nostril.
10. Repeat steps 3 through 8 so you do both nostrils twice.

43 ✺ Sleep

Yoga fails through overexertion.

Hatha Yoga Pradipika 1.15

Sleep is sometimes thought of as an indulgence, a sign of laziness. It is a necessary foundation of health. It is one of the most supportive, restorative, and nurturing practices we can do for our health, our mood, our lives, and our meditation practice.

In Western culture, with its demands on our time, sleep is one of the first things we give up. If we get a full night's sleep, it enhances our clarity of mind, the energy in our body, and our ability to be present without distraction.

If we are sleep-deprived it makes it difficult to meditate. If we don't get a full night's sleep, sitting comfortably with our eyes closed and not getting drowsy becomes a challenge. Trying to focus our internal perceptions is difficult enough without having to fight off sleep.

Even the Dalai Lama is a big proponent of sleep. He says that getting a full night's sleep will make your "daytime calm, relaxed."[1]

So what is a full night's sleep? It is different from person to person. Most of us try to get by on as little sleep as we can, rather than what we need. The average amount of sleep most people need is eight hours. Some need more, some need less, but it's a good place to start.

When you have a couple of days off, let yourself sleep until you feel refreshed. Since you may be catching up on missed sleep, it may take a few nights in a row to get a good idea of how many hours you need. If you wake up with a start, or worrying, give yourself permission to go back to sleep.

You may have trained yourself to wake up at a specific time every day. It may take a while to get past waking up at a set, habitual time.

As we are falling asleep it takes about twenty minutes to settle down through various levels of relaxation. Waking up naturally means coming back up through those levels at our own speed. We surface into consciousness then doze off again, resurface, then doze for shorter and shorter periods of time until we come fully awake. Compare that with having your sleep cycle interrupted by being jolted awake by an alarm clock.

If we wake up at our own natural rate, we spend time in a state that is between sleep and wakefulness. This has been shown to be one of the levels of consciousness that is optimal for activity in the right brain, making the probability of insightful or creative thinking very high.

When you are back on your regular daily schedule, it's important to allow yourself the time to wake up at your own rate. Once you have figured out how many hours you need, set a bedtime that will allow you to wake up naturally. There always seems to be one more thing to do before we go to sleep, one more TV show to watch, one more chapter to read, or one more chore to do. Make your bedtime a priority. Once it's set stick to it.

Just as it is important to have a sacred space for our meditation, it is also important to have a place dedicated only to sleeping and intimacy. Make your bedroom distraction free. Keeping televisions, cell phones, and computers out of the bedroom allows us to attend fully to the importance of our sleep and relationship.

Take sleep on as a real practice, with the same dedication, time commitment, and joyful anticipation that you have for other practices in your life. You will be amazed at what a difference it makes to allow yourself to wake up relaxed and ready for your day. Give yourself the gift of sleep.

Krishnamacharya states the benefits of getting enough sleep most clearly. "Physical health, enthusiasm and liveliness are all benefits of sleep . . . Our body and mind are rejuvenated as a result of sleep . . . One who has not had proper sleep for some time is closer to death."[2]

✳ *The Practice of Sleep*

1. Discover how much sleep you really need, not how much you can get by on.

2. Set a bedtime that will allow you to sleep deeply and wake naturally.

3. Make your bedroom distraction free.

4. Stick to your bedtime.

5. If you wake up prematurely with worries or expectations about your day, give yourself permission to go back to sleep.

6. Take sleep on as a dedicated practice.

44 ✳ Invocation

Practice should be done as learned from your teacher.
HATHA YOGA PRADIPIKA 1.14

Invocation is a way to bring into the present teachers who have taught us our practice or influenced our lives. A true teacher will change our way of thinking, give us a foundation for our practice, and inspire us on the journey to better ourselves. Invoking our teachers can be a way of showing respect. It can be a way of asking for guidance. It can be a way of surrendering to their teaching, their lineage, and the practice they teach.

If given with sincerity, love, and respect, a short prayer said at the beginning of practice can be a powerful tool. Its purpose is to invoke in us, with humility, those attributes that a great teacher possesses.

A Prayer for Help and Guidance
Oh My Teachers,
With love and respect, I touch your feet, and those of
*   your lineage before you.*
Thank you for your patience, wisdom, kindness, and
*   generosity.*

Oh My Teachers,
Help me transform pain into beauty, loss into love,
fear into compassion, sadness into joy, darkness into
*   light, demons into celestial beings.*

Oh My Teachers,
Open my heart and let the divine flow through me.
Let its sound be so beautiful it will change the lives of
*   those who hear it.*
Let its vibration rise in them, giving them peace and
*   awakening love in their heart.*

Oh My Teachers,
Move me from thought and feeling into action, from
*   action into pure sound,*
from pure sound into stillness.

Oh My Teachers,
Remind me I don't have much time, but that I must
*   not rush or be impatient.*

Oh My Teachers,
You chose me for a reason. Help me find mastery as you
*   taught it.*
Remind me that I hold your lineage.

Oh My Teachers,
Though I may struggle and fail, please help me
*   remember that there is only*
one answer: practice.

Oh My Teachers,
Thank you for your teaching. May your name and
*   lineage live on for many generations!*

45 ✸ Lifestyle

It's really outta sight here. It didn't rain. No buttons to push. Right now I'd like to dedicate this song to everybody here with hearts, any kinda hearts and ears.

JIMI HENDRIX, MONTEREY, CA, 1967

JUNK FOOD, DRUGS, AND ROCK AND ROLL

In 1974 I was living the life of a musician. I spent an inordinate amount of time in clubs both playing and listening to music. This of course was accompanied by a more than recreational amount of drinking and drugs. I got sick. During my illness I went through a kind of catharsis. I decided I was no longer going to drink or take drugs. I also decided that I was going to clean up my diet. I was going to start eating healthier food and stop eating animals and animal products.

When I had been in college in Vermont two years earlier, I'd lived in a small house way up in the woods. Knowing that I wouldn't be able to drive in and out after the snow came, I laid in my winter provisions. They consisted of just two items: twelve cases of beer and all the meat I could fit in the freezer. So, this decision to become a sober vegan (which I pronounced *vagen* at the time) was a radical move for me from one end of the lifestyle spectrum to the other. It wasn't easy to do at the time. Not many restaurants or stores offered fare that fit the restrictions of my diet. There was also constant pressure from some of my friends and family, who had shared my previous lifestyle of indulgences, to "loosen up and live a little."

Perhaps I was just replacing one set of obsessive behaviors with another. Perhaps there was a bit of self-flagellation in all of the rules I imposed on myself.

But, has living without eating animals and living without alcohol and drugs helped my meditation practice? Absolutely! I'm still here to meditate, which would have been an open question had I continued on the path I was on. Sadly, many of the musicians I came up with are no longer here.

My mind is probably clearer and more resilient than it would have been had I survived maintaining my old way of life. And at sixty-four, on a good day, I can still get both feet behind my head.

PART NINE

A Final Piece

46 ✳ Innervision

Wherever you are is the entry point.

KABIR

The word *lakshya* means target, aim, goal, or point of attention. It is also a form of Innervision.

The sushumna nadi, the center channel, runs from the root chakra, at the perineum, up the front of the spine to the crown chakra at the top of the head. Bringing the prana up the sushumna from the base of the spine to the top of the head is one of the targets of our Innervision.

The work we have done on bandhas and breath in chapter 34, "Six Additions," and the work we have done on asana, pranayama, and the chakras in part eight ("Supportive and Ancillary Practices"), all turn our attention to raising the prana to the crown chakra.

A blissful loving heart is also a target of our Innervision. We cultivated unconditional love in chapter 26 ("All You Need is Love"), by recalling a time when we either gave or received love without question or expectation of reciprocation.

Another target of our Innervision is the light between the eyebrows. We began to develop this capability by learning where to look, how to look, and what we might see in chapter 27, "The Light." We focused our Innervision to see clouds of transparent green or aquamarine blue light. With practice an indigo "blue pearl" surrounded by a golden saffron corona flaring out from it became visible. With our Innervision we cultivated the ability to see a vast pale horizon before dawn, a bright

160

ball of white light with yellow flames leaping out, and other manifestations of light.

In chapter 29, "The Sound," we learned how to focus our listening, the kinds of sounds we might hear in the nada, and where to listen for them.

These were all points of attention for our Innervision. They are targets that we turn inward to perceive. The final step in each was to reabsorb with each of these lakshyas.

By doing so we open the possibility of the next level of absorption, which is with the *vyoma*. The literal translation of *vyoma* is "sky." In this case it is the internal sky we perceive with our Innervision. This possibility moves us beyond the light of the Inner Divine Light and the Inner Sacred Sound.

The vyoma is subdivided into the five akashas, *akasha* meaning "empty radiant space" or "ether." The five akashas are remarkably similar to the Eight Steps into Clear Light meditation from the *Tibetan Book of the Dead,* which is the subject of the next chapter. Some of the attributes of the akashas that are described in two of the Yoga Upanishads, are exactly the same as those contained in this Buddhist meditation. The five akashas are: a pure empty sky (akasha), a shining black sky (*paraakasha*), an infinite fiery sky (*mahakasha*), a sky brightened by 100,000 unseen suns (*suryakasha*), and the sky of Universal Consciousness (*tattvamakasha*). Smoke, stars, firefly, lamp flame, and moon are also mentioned. Many of these images from the yogic texts overlap with those from "The Eight Steps into Clear Light."

47 ✸ The Eight Steps into Clear Light

*Go, go, go beyond, go beyond beyond. Awaken on the far
shore in enlightenment.*

THE HEART SUTRA

On a beautiful day in May 2007 my dear friend Jonji Provenzano
knocked on my front door. It was unlike him to show up without calling me first. He came in and, in his usual direct way, told me he had
been to the doctor that day and had been diagnosed with terminal
stomach cancer. He had twelve to eighteen months to live. Although
radiation and chemo were both options, surgery was not, due to the
advanced stage of the cancer.

This kind of cancer often goes undetected until its later stages
because the symptoms are minor and could be mistaken for heartburn
or acid-reflux. This is exactly what had happened to Jonji.

I was absolutely dumbstruck. Jonji was my best friend. We had
known one another for more than fifteen years. He had been one of
my first yoga teachers during the 1990s. It was he who'd directed me
toward ashtanga yoga. He had spent more than five years as a member
of my vocal group, Prana. We also had a small study group with another
friend. We would meet anywhere from once a week to once a month
depending on who was going through what life crisis. Jonji and I were
also dharma buddies. We had nurtured and supported one another in
our mutual interests in spirituality.

His diagnosis was particularly difficult because he had just come to a place of true contentment. He had met and married the love of his life, Suzanne, and settled into a comfortable and stable family life with her and her two children.

Suzanne is not only strong, but also loving and kind. She is a nurse who works daily with the sick and dying. Having the combination of her skills and an extremely compassionate heart made it easy for Jonji to die as he wished: in the quiet of his own home, surrounded by his family and friends.

Writer Jeff Davis said of Jonji, "He was a teacher of yoga, meditation, and heart-centered living. He influenced thousands of yoga practitioners with his grounded, intelligent approach to yoga and to life." His classes were known for their thought-provoking, sometimes humorous, dharma talks.

Being the teacher that he was, Jonji chose to turn his dying process into a learning experience for his students and friends. He shared his process of transition through classes, one-on-one sessions, and a journal on Caring Bridge (www.caringbridge.org).

Jonji encouraged everyone to examine their own mortality and clean up whatever was unresolved in their lives. He taught this by example.

He was a master carpenter. While he was still well enough, although sometimes barely, he worked on the house he and Suzanne owned so she wouldn't have to do much to sell it after he died. When he could no longer work, he gave his tools to friends he knew would use them.

He reconciled with his first son from whom he had been estranged for more than twenty years. He healed the wounds from three prior marriages through mutual forgiveness.

Even when bedridden his first question to his many visitors was always, "So, what's going on with you?" After they had answered he would offer loving and compassionate council, often tempered with humor.

Jonji always had a hilarious sense of humor. As he was dying he used that humor as a weapon of love to shatter people's discomfort, sadness, and fear. After hearing one visitor's particularly long tale of woe he said, "Boy, I'm glad I'm not you," and burst out laughing.

We used to play off of one another's jokes. A standard joke between us was how proud we each were of our humility.

I drove Jonji to see his oncologist to schedule his first chemotherapy. By looking at him you wouldn't have known he was sick. At the time I had a shaved head. As we walked in the entranceway to the doctor's building, he took my elbow, as if to steady me. He was playing off the assumption that, having no hair, I was the one people would think was undergoing chemo. In response I slowed my walk to a shuffle. We stopped clowning before we walked into the office. People did look up though, when our arrival was heralded by his rollicking laughter.

One of the first things Jonji did for me after his diagnosis was to give me the Dalai Lama's CD of the *Tibetan Book of the Dead,* which contains the eight steps of dissolution (I refer to them in the meditation at the end of the chapter as "The Eight Steps into Clear Light"). He asked me to learn them. They are a description of what we experience while dying, both before and after the breath stops.

The members of Prana, all of whom loved Jonji, formed a support group for him and Suzanne. We would meet on Sundays at my house to arrange whatever needed to be done for them. At Jonji's urging we also studied the *Tibetan Book of the Dead.* He attended when he wasn't feeling too ill due to either chemo or the cancer.

We used several different versions of the *Tibetan Book of the Dead* for our studies. One of them was by Robert Thurman, who lives locally. A member of the group was friends with Bob and asked if he would come one Sunday to talk to Jonji and the group. One of the first things Bob asked Jonji was, did he know "The Eight Steps of Dissolution"?

In his teaching of "The Eight Steps of Dissolution," Bob emphasizes that it is not only a good way to prepare for and rehearse our death, but it is also used by advanced meditation practitioners to reach higher states of consciousness.

The Tibetan Buddhists believe that after someone leaves their body they spend forty-nine days in the *bardo,* the space between one incarnation and the next. There are readings from the *Tibetan Book of the Dead* that are to be done by friends and family, both while the person is dying and during the forty-nine days immediately after death. In some cases there are very specific instructions on which days to read certain passages; in other cases it's very open-ended. In the months leading up to Jonji's death, he and I organized what parts should be read by our group at what point while he journeyed thorough the bardo.

During that time I often read him the eight steps. The last day he was conscious we finished the schedule of the readings. After that it was as if he had done his work and was ready to go. From then on, when I read him the eight steps, it was no longer practice. It was instruction to help guide him as he left his body.

Needless to say, the eight steps have become a particularly meaningful meditation for me. I practice it regularly.

THE GREAT LIGHT

At the moment of death, you experience The Great Light.
Can you stand it? Have you prepared yourself to dissolve?
JOSEPH CAMPBELL

Many people who have had near-death experiences have recounted seeing a bright white light. The *Tibetan Book of the Dead* warns of a similar experience in the bardo. Between death and rebirth, there is much confusion. The eight steps practice is to make this process familiar so we will not be afraid. During that time in the bardo we will face an overpowering, brilliant white light. It is important not to turn away in fear or distraction, but to move forward into it.

Tibetan Buddhists believe that the first four steps happen before the breath ceases and the last four afterward.

✵ *The Eight Steps into Clear Light, Meditation*

After preparation take your time in holding each of the images in your mind.

1. **Mirage.** As you look out across a broad open desert plane you see what appears to be water lying on the surface of the sand. You notice that rising above the water are waves of shimmering air. Their roiling motion distorts your view. It is the illusion of water, a mirage.

2. **Smoke.** The mirage dissolves into tendrils of warm, misty smoke, slowly moving through a room. Its whiteness stands out against a dark background.

3. **Sparks.** Out of the smoke sparks emerge, spiraling above an unseen fire, rising in swirling, rotating patterns into a night sky.

4. **Candle Flame.** The sparks converge into a single candle flame, its light a soft brightness. The flame, at first, is flickering, its light wavering in the darkness around it. It then becomes still, its light steady, its emanation unwavering.

5. **Moonlit Sky.** The candle flame expands into an open, luminous moonlit sky. The moon is not visible, only its calm, pure white light, suffusing a vast, cloudless sky.

6. **Sunlit Sky.** The moonlit sky dawns into a vivid, hot, red-orange sky lit by the explosive radiant brightness of 100,000 unseen suns.

7. **Black Sky.** Night falls from the sunlit sky to the pitch black darkness after dusk. The vast starless night sky is a bright and glowing blackness. It then darkens even further, to a thick brilliant shining black void.

8. **Clear Light.** The dark night sky then lightens into the transparent clarity of a dawn sky before sunrise. It is a diamond-clear, glass-like light, calming and peaceful. It is an infinite number of imperceptible mirrors reflecting, refracting, and connecting unending light and space.

Return. Return from Clear Light through black darkness, red-orange sunlight, white moonlight, candle flame, sparks, smoke, and mirage back into your body.

❀ *The Eight Steps into Clear Light,*
Advanced Meditation

First, become fluent with these eight steps as visualizations to hold in your mind. Second, think of them not only as visuals, but as environments you are surrounded by and immersed in. Finally, become each of the images of the eight steps in turn.

1. See the mirage. Be in the mirage. Co-absorb with the mirage.
2. See the smoke. Be in the smoke. Co-absorb with the smoke.
3. See the sparks. Be in the sparks. Co-absorb with the sparks.
4. See the candle flame. Be in the candle flame. Co-absorb with the candle flame.
5. See the moonlit sky. Be in the moonlit sky. Co-absorb with the moonlit sky.
6. See the sunlit sky. Be in the sunlit sky. Co-absorb with the sunlit sky.
7. See the black sky. Be in the black sky. Co-absorb with the black sky.
8. See the Clear Light. Be in the Clear Light. Become the Clear Light.
9. Return through all of these steps in reverse order back into your body.

48 ✸ Practice, Practice, Practice!

Balance and prayer are self-confrontational. Behind the muscular and spiritual exertion there must be a point of effortless calm. At that point you meet yourself.

PETER HØEG

In paragliding you lift off the side of a mountain, using only the power of the wind to fly an elliptical-shaped parachute or "wing." You soar like a bird on rising currents of warm air.

As you are learning how to fly, you are taught the phrase "target fixation." It means, if you don't want to fly into the tree, don't look at the tree.

If you are coming in for a landing and there is a tree at the edge of the landing area, don't look at it. Even though you may be using all of your strength to steer away from it, if your attention is fixed on it, you will fly into the tree. Look where you want to land, not where you don't want to land. In life we move toward what we focus on, even if it's something we don't want. We become what we pay attention to.

Our brain is highly adaptable in its ability to learn. Neuroplasticity is the ability to rewire the brain to learn new skills or to compensate for a brain injury. Changes in the brain aren't restricted to just rerouting neural pathways, it is also possible to change the thickness of the gray matter and the actual physical shape of the brain.

There is a correlation between the development of a specific practice or skill and the thickening of a specific area of the cerebral cortex. There is a marked increase in the thickness of gray matter in athletes in the motor areas of the brain, in musicians in the music areas of the brain, and in multilingual people in the language areas of the brain.

Dr. Sara Lazar, who teaches at Harvard School of Medicine, did a clinical study to measure if regular meditation practice over time would change the brain physically. The study found that four regions in the brain used in meditation grew thicker in participants who meditated. The members of the control group who did not meditate showed no change in gray matter. The study also concluded that the longer you cultivated a meditation practice, the thicker one specific area of the brain grew.

The study states that meditation "is associated with changes in gray matter concentration in brain regions involved in learning and memory processes, emotion regulation, self-referential processing, and perspective taking."[1]

In addition the study found that regular meditation slows the thinning of the cerebral cortex that normally takes place with aging.

We know that when we do yoga, the practice changes our body. We stretch and become more flexible. We build muscle and become stronger. Recent studies have shown that when we meditate on breath, image, and sound, the practice changes our brain. It causes changes in both the neuroplasticity and the physical structure of our brain. We now have scientific proof that every time we sit in meditation, we are rewiring and rebuilding our brain.

We can only benefit from meditation if we do the practice. We can read about it, think about it, talk about it, but unless we do the practice, there is no opportunity to have the experiences that will transform us. This must be sustained, as the *Yoga Sutras* say, "with devotion, through time."

Of course, sometimes life intercedes and makes it impossible to practice. It is often the first thing we give up when we need it the most.

Don't beat up on yourself about missing a practice. Let it make your resolve even stronger that you will get back to the meditation cushion as soon as possible.

This practice is simple. That doesn't mean it's easy. It is always possible to come up with a reason not to practice. On the other hand, it is not impossible to come up with a reason *to* practice. You may have to give something up. You may need to sacrifice something in order to sit down and meditate. That is part of the practice as well. The practice of practicing is a practice.

✸ Practice

1. Go and sit on your meditation cushion.

IN OR OUT?

There is so much flickering bright light and noise in our culture to distract us. They pull us away from the divine, the divine within us that is connected to the divine in everything. We only have a limited amount of time here. Life is short. Which will you chose? Where will you put your attention? What will you become?

I had the opportunity to briefly meet A. G. Mohan, a wonderful teacher who was a student of T. Krishnamacharya for twenty years. Krishnamacharya was also teacher to Sri K. Pattabhi Jois, B. K. S. Iyengar, and T. K. V. Desikachar, among many others. When I asked Mohan about my experiences with this practice, his response was, "The taste is in the pudding." In other words, if the practice gives you benefit, brings you peace, and contentment, if it changes your life for the better, then there is no question, do it!

CLOSING

In closing we return back to where we first began: the idea that everything is vibrating. Each vibration, each sound, has a place in the

Universal Orchestra creating one unified sound. This sound, the nada, has no beginning or end. It is everywhere enlivening everything. We are all part of it and it is all part of us. We are one with the One.

✸ *The Sound of the Universal Meditation*

1. What is the sound of total relaxation?
2. What is the sound of absolute truth?
3. What is the sound of overwhelming beauty?
4. What is the sound of complete compassion?
5. What is the sound of unconditional love?
6. What is the sound of joyful bliss?
7. What is the sound of the Universe?
8. What would you hear if you could listen through God's ears?

Gratitude

I would like to thank my guru, Sri K. Pattabhi Jois, for teaching the practice of ashtanga yoga. I studied with him from 2000 until 2008, both here in the United States and in Mysore, India. I feel fortunate to have had that time with him. The impact of his teaching changed my life. It is a practice that I begin anew every morning when I step on the mat. It changes my body. It lifts my spirit. It informs every note of my music.

My daily practice, although dedicated and regular, is not advanced or completely correct. Nonetheless, I would not have written this book, be making the music I do, or have the life I have were it not for him. I realize that at the heart of whatever small success I have is Guruji and his teaching. My gratitude is unending.

During my first visit to Mysore, after practice one day, he said to me, "You perfect." Not being able to take in what I had heard, I said, "Excuse me?" He said, "Today, you perfect." I know he wasn't talking about my asana practice, which was far from perfect. He was talking about that part of all of us that is perfect. I had often heard him say, "God is in everything." At that moment I understood that each of us is part of that "everything."

On those days when I struggle in either my practice or my life, I remember his words, "Today you perfect" (as we all are), and I smile.

Acknowledgments

My deepest thanks to:

Eddie Stern, who took the time to sit with me and read through the verses of the *Hatha Yoga Pradipika*. His insight and knowledge of yoga were of exceptional help to me in the writing of this book. Since 1999 I have had the good fortune to be his ashtanga yoga student when I am in New York City.

Shubhraji, with whom I have studied Vedanta since 1999. Her guidance and encouragement, both in my life and in writing this book, have been of extraordinary value to me. Her teachings on Vedanta helped shape this book.

Robert Thurman, to whom I will be forever grateful, for taking the time to come talk to my dear friend Jonji and his support group as Jonji was dying of cancer. Jonji was overjoyed by Bob's visit that afternoon. I have taken yearly teachings with Bob on the relationship between Buddha and the yogis since 2006. The meditation on the Eight Steps into Clear Light is based to some degree on his instruction.

His Holiness the Dalai Lama, whom I have had the privilege of hearing teach yearly from 2006 to 2010. He is a beacon of light for those who believe that love, kindness, and compassion are the most powerful forces known to mankind.

Krishna Das, for all of his generosity in sharing his music and the stage with me and Prana since 2005 and for the foreword he contributed to this book. I have great respect for him both as a kirtan wallah and a person.

Eric, Joncarl, and Katina Hersey, my children, who have all in their own ways taught me about unconditional love. Although I can take very little responsibility for who they are becoming, they are the best reason I have for being here on this Earth.

Gina Dominique, for her love and support: an enduring light in my life. With her every chapter is more surprising, exciting, and fulfilling than the last.

John Hersey, my father, who was a kind, compassionate, thoughtful, and ethical man. He has been a true role model for me.

Frances Ann Cannon, my mother, who encouraged my interest in music. She bought me records, took me to concerts and Broadway musicals, and arranged music lessons for me. These acts of recognition and kindness helped shape me and my life.

Ann, Brook, Martin, and John Hersey, my sisters and brothers, who, each in their own unique way, have influenced the direction of my life.

Tom Guralnick, my lifelong friend, who has supported my music no matter what twist or turn it has taken.

The members of Prana, who have shown up at my house on almost every Monday night since 2000 to sing my music. Among them: Peter Buettner, Amy Fradon, Kirsti Gholson, Julie Last, Bruce Milner, Julian Lines, Leslie Ritter, Joe Veillette, Amy Goldin, Julie Parisi, and Bar Scott.

Robert (Rick) Bartz, D.C., who generously shared his broad knowledge of physiology and anatomy in answer to my many questions as I wrote this book. Thanks to him and all of the other ashtanga yogis who have shown up at my house, week after week, year after year, to join me in self-practice.

Mark Kinder, for some illuminating thoughts on sound and light meditations.

Ruth Levine, who for many years encouraged me to write and offered me many insightful observations.

Marcia Albert, my first yoga teacher, who with love and deep knowledge started me on this path of yoga and sound.

Teachers through the years have included: Sharath Rangaswamy Jois, Saraswathi Rangaswamy Jois, Manju Jois, Jerry Bidlack, Alvin Lucie, Bill Dixon, Henry Brant, Jane Odin, Bobby McFerrin, Beryl and Thom Birch, David Swenson, Nancy Gilgoff, Barbara Boris, David Hykes, Lobsang Phuntsok, Tim Miller, Richard Freeman, Odsuren Baatar, Made and Suathi Bandem, and Alash.

Martin Barding, for his photography, both here in this book and all the photos he has taken of Prana over the years.

Mavis Gewant, for her contribution of the lovely illustration in this book.

Kathy McNames of Yoga Vermont and Francois Raoult of Sky Yoga, for their ongoing support of my teaching over the years.

Ned Leavitt, for his insightful instruction on the publishing world and contract negotiation.

Jeff Davis, for his willingness to point me where I needed to go.

Robin Bourjaily, for her excellent and insightful copyediting.

Jon Graham, Jamaica Burns, Jeanie Levitan, Virginia Scott Bowman, Priscilla Baker, Manzanita Carpenter, Erica B. Robinson, Kelly Bowen, and all of the staff at Inner Traditions, especially Ehud and Vatsala Sperling.

A. G. Mohan, who, although I only met him briefly, communicated to me that I was on the right path.

The Source Texts

I have included in this appendix those verses that are relevant to the practice of nada yoga. Since this is an experiential practice rather than an intellectual one, I have avoided technical language with its deeper and often diffuse meanings. I have tried to present these texts, rather than in their literal translations, in language that is accessible and easily understood as instruction. In some cases I have only included what is pertinent to the daily practice.

This practice is primarily drawn from the second half of the fourth chapter of the *Hatha Yoga Pradipika*. I also use verses from the *Yoga Sutras* to support and elucidate the primary teaching. In addition I have drawn on verses from the *Chandogya Upanishad, Rig-Veda, Adidaivat Pratipaadhak Khand, Goraksha Paddhati, Siddha Siddanta Paddhati, Goraksha Shataka, Yoga Kundalini Upanishad, Advaya Taraka Upanishad, Mandukya Upanishad, Narada Parivrajaka Upanishad, Yoga Taravali, Gheranda Samhita, Shiva Sutras, Shiva Samhita, Amitra Bindu Upanishad, Amitra Nada Bindu Upanishad, Hamsa Upanishad,* and *Srimad Bhagavatam* to broaden or cross-correlate some of the instructions for meditation put forth in the *Hatha Yoga Pradipika* and *Yoga Sutras.*

CHANDOGYA UPANISHAD

The *Chandogya Upanishad* is one of the earliest of the 108 Upanishads, a seminal teaching from the Vedic Age (approx. 1500–500 BCE). It contains the most important verse of the *Advaita* (non-dualist) school of Vedanta.

> 6.8.7. *"You are that." ("Tat tvam asi.") The individual Divine Self (Atman) and the Universal Consciousness (Brahman) are one and the same.*

In all of the texts that follow, the word *Reality* is used to express this concept of Oneness.

RIG-VEDA

The *Rig-Veda* is a set of Indian verses in Sanskrit. Three-and-a-half millennia old, it is one of the world's oldest religious texts.

> 1.164.45. *There are four levels of speech, the spiritually wise know them all. Three are secret. Mortals use the fourth.*

ADIDAIVAT PRATIPAADHAK KHAND

The *Adidaivat Pratipaadhak Khand* is from the *Ganapati Atharvasirsha Upanishad* that dates from the sixteenth or seventeenth century.

> 5.6. *You (Lord Ganesha) are the four levels of speech: para, pashyanti, madhyama and vaikhari.*

HATHA YOGA PRADIPIKA

The *Hatha Yoga Pradipika* can be translated as "Light on Yoga" or "The Great Lamp of Yoga." It is a collection of Vedic texts on yoga gathered by Swami Svatmarama. The section that deals with nada yoga (4.65–4.102) is attributed to his teacher, Gorakshanath. A large part of this teaching is taken from the *Goraksha Paddhati* that is derived from the *Nada-Bindu Upanishads*, part of the *Rig-Veda*.

Gorakshanath was a sage and teacher who lived from the eleventh into the twelfth century CE. He traveled throughout India and neighboring countries. His many writings collated, codified, and evolved the practices of yoga, among them nada yoga. Gorakshanath was a disciple of Matsyendranath, the founder of the Nath lineage. Gorakshanath's writings and teaching had a great impact on that lineage. He is held, by some, in the same high regard as Sankara, Patanjali, Buddha, and Shiva.

The *Hatha Yoga Pradipika* usually consists of four chapters, although there are versions with five. The chapters divide hatha yoga into lessons on distinctive practices. These are: asana (postures), pranayama (breath control), mudra (physical or mental "gesture"), and samadhi (realization, reabsorption). The second half of the chapter on samadhi is a teaching on nada yoga.

The verses on nada yoga in the *Hatha Yoga Pradipika* give us simple, practical, easy-to-follow instructions on listening for, hearing, and maintaining a connection with the Inner Sacred Sound. You need not be a learned master or even a student of yoga to progress in the practice of nada yoga. It is developed and deepened through regular and dedicated practice in sitting meditation.

1.14. *Practice should be done as learned from your teacher.*

1.15. *Yoga fails through overexertion.*

1.35. *Sit in siddhasana by pressing the perineum with the left heal. Place the other heel on the pubic bone. Fix the gaze between the eyebrows.*

1.37. *Siddhasana is also called "muktasana."*

1.43. *There is no other laya (absorption), which equals the nada (internal sound).*

1.46. *Place the tongue on the root of the top front teeth.*

2.30. *Neti purifies the head, gives divine sight, and destroys disease above the shoulders.*

3.55. *Uddiyanabandha binds the prana and causes it to "fly up" the sushumna (center channel).*

3.57. Uddiyanabandha is pulling the belly in and the navel up.

3.61. Mula bandha is pressing the heel on the perineum and contracting the anus causing the apana (downward prana) to move upward through the sushumna (center channel).

3.64. When the practice of mula bandha brings together prana/apana and nada/bindu, yoga (union) is reached.

4.10. The practice of asana, pranayama, and mudras wakes up the kundalini, and prana is absorbed in the sushumna (center channel).

4.29. The senses are ruled by the mind. The mind is ruled by the breath. The breath is ruled by absorption in the nada.

4.32. When there is stillness in body and mind, indescribable bliss arises.

4.36. Shambhavimudra is a one-pointed inward focus while gazing as if looking outward.

4.37. When mind (consciousness) and breath (prana) are absorbed in the internal light with a fixed gaze, this is the attainment of Reality.

4.39. Fixing the pupils on the light causes samadhi.

4.41. In shambhavimudra, one's still mind attains the form of the eternal radiant light which illuminates All.

4.56. Empty inside, empty outside, empty like a pot in air. Full inside, full outside, full like a pot in the ocean.

4.57. Don't have a single thought. Let all of them go, both thoughts of the external and the internal.

4.58. The entire universe is just a projection of the mind. The play of our thoughts is just a projection of mind.

4.65. Here now begins the teaching of nada yoga as taught by Gorakshanath, accessible to all, even those with no experience of yoga.

4.66. Hearing the nada is the most important of all meditative absorptions.

4.67. In muktasana, and holding shambhavimudra, listen

*with one-pointedness to the sound of the nada within the
right ear.*

4.68. *A clear distinct sound is heard in the sushumna (center
channel) when the ears, eyes, mouth, and nose are closed.*

4.70. *When anahata chakra is penetrated, the nada is a
blissful feeling like polyphonic tinkling vibrating in the
body.*

4.72 & 4.73. *Then, the prana unites from the ida and pingala
nadis (side channels) and enters the vishuddha chakra and
there is a blissful feeling above the soft palate, and sound of
a low drum, or conch shell.*

4.74 & 4.75. *Then, the prana rises to the ajna chakra. In that
space the beating of a drum is heard. Being beyond thought,
the Supreme Bliss arises.*

4.76 & 4.78. *Prana passes through ajna chakra and rises
to the sahasrara chakra. There is the sound of a flute.
"Reality" is attained. This is raja yoga.*

4.80. *Meditating between the brows quickly brings samadhi.*

4.81. *Indescribable bliss arises in the heart of the yogi who
meditates on the nada.*

4.82. *Close both the ears . . . and listen to the sound until the
mind becomes steady.*

4.83. *Practicing this sound meditation diminishes exterior
sounds. Through listening to the nada for fifteen days the
yogi overcomes all obstacles and feels blissful.*

4.84, 4.85, & 4.86. *Loud sounds are initially heard. Subtler
ones are heard as practice grows . . . the ocean, thunder, a
large waterfall, low drums, large bell, conch shell, horn,
flute, tinkling chimes, bees, or crickets.*

4.87. *After hearing the loud sounds, fix the mind on the
subtlest of the subtle sounds.*

4.88. *Keep the mind steady on the nada, even when it moves
from the gross to the subtle or from the subtle to the gross.*

4.89. *Whatever sound the mind is drawn to, settle on it, adhere to it, and become absorbed in it.*

4.93. *One who desires true union of yoga should leave all thinking behind and concentrate with single-pointed attention on the nada.*

4.100. *The mind redissolves into the Inner Sacred Sound and the Internal Divine Light, and they are again recognized as one.*

4.101. *Reabsorption goes beyond sound. Without sound there is no space, only the Ultimate Reality.*

4.102. *The sound of nada is shakti (or Brahman), formlessness in which all else dissolves, Reality. Here ends the teaching on the nada.*

GORAKSHA PADDHATI

I have only included here the relevant verses that are not included in the *Hatha Yoga Pardipika*.

1.72. *The bindhu is located in the soft palate ("bell," uvula).*

1.85. *Om is the Divine Light. A-U-M. The m is the bindu.*

2.15. *When the all-pervasive Divine Light is seen, all karma stops.*

2.35. *The three natures (tamas, rajas, and sattva) are released when the anahata (unstruck) sound is heard in the heart.*

2.71. *Controlling prana and focusing the gaze between the eyebrows will manifest the nila bindu (blue light).*

2.73. *Meditate between the brows to hear the Inner Sacred Sound.*

SIDDHA SIDDANTA PADDHATI

Another text by Gorakshanath.

2. *A yogi knows the nine chakras. (The two additional chakras*

*are: the talu chakra at the root of the soft palate and the
akasha chakra at the very top of the head.)*

*At the third chakra (manipura), a subtle continuous nada is
heard.*

*At the fourth chakra (anahata), a luminous light (jyotis rupa)
shines.*

*At the fifth chakra (vishuddha), a powerful continuous nada
is heard.*

*Between the eyebrows, at the eye of wisdom, a steady thumb-
sized flame burns.*

*A yogi knows the three inner vision targets (tri-lakshyas). They
are internal (antar lakshya), external (bahir lakshya), and
the middle (madhya lakshya).*

GORAKSHA SHATAKA

Also written by Gorakshanath.

*Meditate on the body as a house supported by one column
(the spine). It has nine doors to the external world (eyes, ears,
nostrils, mouth, genitals, and anus). Prana flows through the
nine main nadis to them. The tenth door is at the root of the
palate and opens upward to the Divine.*

YOGA SUTRAS

Patanjali was a sage and grammarian who lived sometime around
the second century BCE. In the *Yoga Sutras*, he gathered a series of
concise statements that instruct and illustrate the deeper truths of yoga.
They are a codification into one of many schools of teaching on the
unfoldment of raja yoga.

1.2. Yoga is stilling the distraction in the mind.

*1.14. Practice is the foundation of stillness when sustained
with devotion through time.*

1.27. *Through the sound Om we see the reflection of our own true nature.*

1.29. *Its repetition removes all obstacles and reveals the inner self.*

1.36. *Meditation on the blissful light within brings the mind to stillness.*

1.38. *Recalling the dream state or deep sleep state while in the waking state brings stillness to the mind.*

1.41. *Samadhi is when the observer, observing, and object observed become one and shine with crystal clarity.*

2.28. *Through the practice of the Eight Limbs of Yoga, we are purified, and the Light of Wisdom shows us the difference between illusion and Reality.*

2.29. *Yama, niyama, asana, pranayama, pratyahara, dharana, dhyana, and samadhi are the eight limbs of yoga.*

2.30. *The yamas are: ahimsa, satya, asteya, brahmacarya, and aparigraha.*

2.32. *The niyamas are: saucha, samtosa, tapas svahyaya, and isvarapranidhanani.*

2.46. *Sitting in stillness with comfort is asana.*

2.47. *Perfection in asana is attained by letting go of effort and meditating on Reality.*

2.49. *Regulating the inhale and exhale of the breath is pranayama.*

2.51. *Effortless pranayama happens when in concentration.*

2.52. *Pranayama lifts the veil of ignorance from the Inner Light.*

2.54. *When the organs of the senses are withdrawn from external distractions and perception is directed inward, this is pratyahara.*

3.1. *Placing the attention on one point is dharana.*

3.2. *Dhyana is an uninterrupted, stable stream of concentration on one point.*

3.3. *When all else appears empty, and the "observer" is enveloped by the object, and they become one, this is samadhi.*

3.4. *The continuum of dharana, dhyana, and samadhi, directed to an object, is samyama.*

3.26. *Samyama on the light within, to reveal the subtle, veiled, and distant.*

3.33. *Meditate on the light at the crown of the head (sahasrara chakra) to bring visions of masters and celestial beings.*

3.34. *When the light is seen, even if suddenly, all is known.*

3.35. *Meditate on the heart (anahata chakra) to understand the mind (consciousness).*

3.42. *Hearing with a divine ear is attained by contemplation of the relationship of space and sound.*

THE YOGA UPANISHADS

These are all part of the Yoga Upanishads, a collection of twenty teachings from different time periods, diverse locations, and many yogic traditions. Their emphasis is on specific instruction of a variety of yogic practices.

Yoga Kundalini Upanishad

18 & 19. *The power of speech in its seed form, para, sprouts up in the muladhara chakra. It grows into leaves, pashyanti, in the anahta chakra, becomes a bud, madhyama, in the vishuddha chakra, and blossoms, vaikhari, in the throat. When taken in the reverse order, the sound reaches absorption.*

20 & 21. *Whoever rests in "I am He" remains in equilibrium, unaffected by high or low words spoken to them.*

Mandala Brahman Upanishad

1.1.2–11. *The eight limbs of yoga are: yamas, niyamas, asana, pranayama, pratyahara, dharana, dhyana, and samadhi. He who knows this, knows Reality.*

1.2.5. *Turning the Innervision on the tri lakshya (three forms of targets), antar lakshya (external), bahir lakshya (internal), and madhya lakshya (middle) brings the yogi to Reality.*

1.2.6. *The yogi should fix the Innervision on the antar lakshya (internal target), of the prana, burning brightly as it rises from the root chakra (muladhara) to the crown chakra (sahasrara) through the center channel (sushumna nadi). It is as powerful as lightning and as subtle as a thread in a lotus stem. It removes the darkness that covers ignorance (avidya). By seeing it in the abiding place of the supreme consciousness (Bhramara Guha).*

1.2.7. *By closing the ears and fixing his attention on the hissing of the nada, the yogi reabsorbs with the sound and sees, between the eyes, the blue light (nila-jyoti), which also illuminates the heart.*

1.2.8. *By fixing the Innervision on the bahir lakshya (external targets), he sees light the color of blue water, and indigo surrounded by gold and red/yellow, between four and twelve finger-widths (angulas) in front of the nose.*

1.2.10. *When the yogi sees a bright spiritual light (jyoti) twelve finger-widths (angulas) above the crown chakra (sahasrara), bliss arises.*

1.2.11. *With the Innervision fixed on the madhya lakshya (middle targets) the yogi sees and absorbs with a vast expansive horizon at dawn. It is colored by the Sun, the Moon, a blazing fire, none of which can be seen.*

1.2.12–1.2.14. *With constant practice he reabsorbs into akasha (a pure empty sky), paraakasha (a shining black*

sky), mahakasha (an infinite fiery sky), suryakasha (a
sky brightened by 100,000 unseen suns), and finally he
reabsorbs into tattvamakasha (Universal Consciousness).

2.1.10. When meditation is practiced on lakshya (the targets of
Innervison), the yogi sees a unending sphere of light which
is Universal Consciousness.

2.2.1. Then the crystal, smoke, stars, firefly, lamp flame, eye,
and gold are seen.

2.5.2. Yoga nidra (the sleep of the yogi) brings the infinite bliss
of Universal Consciousness.

Advaya Taraka Upanishad

2. With the eyes completely shut or slightly open, look inward
above the middle of the eyebrows to see the Supreme Light
of Universal Consciousness, and thereby know Reality.

4. Meditate on the tri-lakshya (three Innervision targets) to
attain Universal Consciousness.

5. The antar lakshya (internal targets) of the Innervision are
the lightning-bright kundalini rising through the sushumna
to the top of the head, the effluent light shining brilliantly
in the center of the forehead, the hissing of the nada, and
the nila bindu (blue light) between the eyes to see. Seeing
these will cause bliss to arise in the heart.

6. The bahir lakshya (external targets of the Innervision) are
rays of brilliant yellow, blood-red, and radiant blue light.
As the focus settles, molten gold is seen at the edge of vision.

7. The madhya lakshya (middle targets of the Innervision) are
vast vistas, like the sky lit by a brilliant burning, unseen
Sun, like the sky lit by a pale unseen Moon, like the clear
morning sky before dawn. When they are internally
perceived and reabsorbed, then one proceeds to perceive and
reabsorb with the five akashas.

10. Turn the mind from "form" (that which the sense organs

*perceive) to the "formless" (internal perception). Meditate
with vision beyond what the physical eye can see to perceive
pure white light. Turn the mind's eye to the point within
the heart where the light of the Divine Self burns.*

11. *Look between the eyebrows at the internal light. Co-absorb
with it. Meditate on the light above the palate.*

13. *The internal light is the ultimate embodiment of Reality. It
resides in the higher consciousness, the radiant blossoming of
the thousand-petaled lotus at the crown of the skull, and a
point sixteen angulas (finger-widths) above the top of the head.*

Amitra Bindu Upanishad

11. *The Atman is present in waking, dreaming, and deep sleep.
Rebirth does not occur for those who surpass those three
states.*

16. *Om is the Divine Sound. The sound beyond m is a silent
echo of Om. Meditate on that silence to know Reality.*

Amitra Nada Bindu Upanishad

4. *After sounding Om, abandon the vocal sound and dissolve
into soundless letter m and into the subtlety of the anahata
(unstruck) sound.*

Dhyana Bindu Upanishad

61. *The breath comes out with the sound Hum and goes in with
the sound So, meaning "I Am He."*

Hamsa Upanishad

4. *In a day there are 21,600 breaths.*

Mandukya Upanishad

1. *All is Om. It is the past, present, and future. It is also beyond
the past, present, and future.*

2. *Om is Brahman. Brahman is the Self. The Self exists in four states.*

3. *The first is the Self in the waking state, having consciousness of the exterior world, gross objects.*

4. *The second is the Self in the dreaming state, having consciousness of the interior world, subtle objects.*

5. *The third is the state of deep sleep. There is no desire, no dreams. The Self in deep sleep is blissful unity without conscious awareness. The preceding state is its doorway.*

6. *In the fourth state, turiya, there is no consciousness of the external world, or of the internal world, nor is there unconsciousness. It is the same Self as in all three of the preceding states, but all phenomenon have come to stillness. It is pure consciousness, pure awareness.*

7. *This Self is the letters of Om, A, U, and M.*

8. *The waking state is A.*

9. *The dreaming state is U.*

10. *Deep sleep is M.*

11. *The silence after the sound is the turiya state.*

Narada Parivrajaka Upanishad

9. *While in a body there are the four states: waking, dreaming, deep sleeping, and the turiya state. The ever-present Atman is beyond the first three states.*

SHIVA SUTRAS

The *Shiva Sutras* were composed by Panini who was a Sanskrit grammarian who lived in the fourth century BCE.

1.7. *During waking, dreaming, and deep sleep, the turiya state is present.*

1.8. *In the waking state we perceive the external world through the senses.*

1.9. *In the dreaming state we perceive the internal world through mental activity.*

1.10. *In the deep sleep state there is no perception.*

1.11. *The one who experiences the three states is in control of the senses.*

1.12. *The domain of the union is an astonishment.*

1.6. *In union with the chakras, one withdraws from the universe.*

1.18. *The bliss of divine sight is the joy of samadhi.*

2.2. *Steady practice brings attainment.*

3.15. *By naturally casting the gaze, what is internal is seen as external.*

3.17. *In asana one sinks with comfort into the lake of bliss.*

3.20. *Sound is the source of all beings.*

3.22. *By penetrating internal perceptions one is absorbed in Reality.*

SHIVA SAMHITA

The *Shiva Samhita* is a comprehensive set of verses on all aspects of yoga framed as a teaching by Shiva to Parvati. It was written at the end of the seventeenth, or beginning of the eighteenth, century. Its authorship is not presently known.

5.36 & 5.37. *Closing the ears, eyes, nose, and mouth, the yogi quickly sees the light of the luminous self.*

5.38. *By seeing the light, even for a moment, one becomes pure and blissful.*

5.41. *Meditation on the nada quickly brings the yogi to bliss.*

5.42 & 5.43. *The first sounds are bees and vina, then through practice, a bell and thunder.*

5.44. *If the yogi remains in concentration on the sound, reabsorption occurs.*

5.45. *When the yogi is absorbed in the nada, the external world falls away and bliss arises.*

5.62. *When the yogi meditates on the crown chakra, a brilliant light as bright as lightning is seen.*

5.130. *By meditating on the great light, the yogi becomes enlightened.*

5.144. *At the ajna chakra is the bindu where the prana and shakti come and coalesce as the nada.*

GHERANDA SAMHITA

The *Gheranda Samhita* is another in-depth instructional guide on yoga, as collected by Gheranda at the end of the seventeenth century CE.

2.7. *Sit in siddhasana by pressing the perineum with the left heel. Place the other heel on the pubic bone. Bring the chin to the chest. Sit perfectly still. Turn the senses inward. Look with a steady gaze between the eyebrows. This brings Liberation.*

6.17. *Meditate on the light of the primordial sound between the eyebrows. Join with it in an unbroken stream of luminosity.*

7.7. *Through shambhavimudra, see the self. Fix your attention on the bindu of Reality.*

7.8. *Put the self in the sound and the sound in the self. When the self is sound all else falls away.*

7.10. *Focus on the sound and bliss will come from the attainment of Reality.*

YOGA TARAVALI

Written by Adi Sankara at the beginning of the ninth century, the *Yoga Taravali* is a poem on his teachings on yoga. Although Sankara is best known as the establishing light of *Advaita Vedanta,* he was also a master of yoga.

2. *The highest of all absorptions is nada yoga, from which the highest form of samadhi will arise.*

4. *Precious nada yoga and the power of prana will reabsorb with the anahata chakra and Reality will be reached.*

6. *Jalamdhara bandha, uddiyana bandha, and mula bandha awaken the sleeping kundalini, which enters the sushumna (center channel) and causes the breath to become regular.*

18. *Quieting the breath, senses, and mind, and holding the body in stillness, the yogi becomes dissolved in light like an unflickering lamp.*

21. *The yogi who regulates the breath, stills the body, and looks inward as if looking outward, attains a still mind.*

22. *Comfortably looking inward as if looking outward, letting go of "I" and "mine," regulating the breath, and stilling the mind, the yogi goes to the cave of the heart where only a clear, open, vast sky exists.*

24. *When the seeds of samskaras are burned, and the external world holds no interest, the yogi, in total absorption, appears to be sleeping (yoga nidra).*

25. *With steady practice and the burning of the seeds of all samskaras, the yogi reaches absorption of the highest degree and remains there in yoga nidra.*

27. *When the light of Universal Consciousness shines forth and removes ignorance, the yogi perceives Reality without the play of the world.*

BRAHMA JNANAVALI MALA

Also written by Adi Sankara.

16. *I (the Atman) am the witness of the three states of waking, dreaming, and deep sleep. I am the Self, immortal and unchanging.*

SRIMAD BHAGAVATAM

The *Srimad Bhagavatam* is one of the most important of all Hindu texts. It dates from the ninth to thirteenth centuries CE.

> *11.21.36 & 11.21.37. The transcendental sound perceived by the senses in the mind is unending and is as deep as the ocean. Absolute Reality is manifest in the form of that sound. God's breath is heard in the mind as different sounds.*
>
> *12.6.37 & 12.6.38. His mind quiet, he hears in his heart the subtlest transcendental sound from the ether. That sound can be heard when the ears are blocked from external sound. Devotion to that sound cleanses the heart.*

BARDO THODOL (TIBETAN BOOK OF THE DEAD)

Padmasambhava, who is sometimes called the second Buddha, conceived the *Tibetan Book of the Dead* in the eighth century CE. After its transcription, it was hidden in Tibet until it was found by Karma Lingpa in the twelfth century.

> *Just as you stop breathing, you will see the primal Clear Light.*
> *A mirage is the earth element dissolving into the water element.*
> *Smoke is the water element dissolving into the fire element.*
> *Glowing sparks are the fire element dissolving into the air element.*
> *A white moonlit sky is the space element dissolving into "luminosity."*
> *A red sunlit sky is the "luminosity" dissolving into "brightness."*
> *A black night sky is "brightness" dissolving into "near attainment."*
> *A morning twilight sky is "near attainment" dissolving into "Clear Light."*

Notes

CHAPTER 2. WHAT IS NADA YOGA?

1. Michael, *The Law of Attention*, 11.
2. Khan, *The Mysticism of Sound and Music*, 40.
3. Carrera, *Inside the Yoga Sutras*, 390.
4. Khan, *The Mysticism of Sound and Music*, 41.
5. Muktananda, *Satsang with Baba: Volume 5*, 63.

CHAPTER 20. THE COLORS OF YOUR MIND

1. Ramachandran, "3 Clues to Understanding Your Brain," www.ted.com/talks/vilayanur_ramachandran_on_your_mind.html.

CHAPTER 25. THE POSTURE

1. Sankara, *Yoga Taravali*, 61.
2. Campbell, *Sukhavati*.
3. Bear, Connors, and Paradiso, *Neuroscience: Exploring the Brain*, 604.

CHAPTER 27. THE LIGHT

1. Patanjali, *The Yoga Sutras of Patanjali*, 60.
2. Patanjali, *The Yoga Sutras of Patanjali*, 111.
3. Patanjali, *Light on the Yoga Sutras of Patanjali*, 83.
4. Svatmarama, *The Hatha Yoga Pradipika*, 69.
5. Patanjali, *Yoga Philosophy of Patanjali*, 248.
6. Svatmarama, *Hathapradipika*, 145.
7. Banerjea, *The Philosophy of Gorakhnath with Goraksha Vacana-Sangraha*, 191.

CHAPTER 29. THE SOUND

1. Sarasvati, *Nada Yoga,* 11.

CHAPTER 34. SIX ADDITIONS

1. Stern, "The Practice," http://kpjayi.org/the-practice.

CHAPTER 39. PRANAYAMA

1. Desikachar, *The Heart of Yoga,* 181.

CHAPTER 43. SLEEP

1. Dalai Lama and Huffington, http://on.aol.com/video/arianna-and-the
   -dalai-lama-discuss-sleep-517365946.
2. Krishnamacharya, *Yoga Makaranda,* intro. 6.

CHAPTER 48. PRACTICE, PRACTICE, PRACTICE!

1. Hölzel et al., "Mindfulness Practice Leads to Increases in Regional Brain
   Gray Matter Density."

Bibliography

Aja. *Mantra: The Power of Sound*. Portland, Ore.: ATMA, 1989.

Banerjea, Akshaya Kumar. *The Philosophy of Gorakhnath with Goraksha Vacana-Sangraha*. Gorakhpur, India: Mahant Dig Vija Nath Trust, 1961.

Beck, Guy L. *Sonic Theology, Hinduism and Sacred Sound*. Columbia, S.C.: University of South Carolina Press, 1993.

Bear, Mark F., Barry W. Connors, and Michael A. Paradiso. *Neuroscience: Exploring the Brain*. 3rd ed. Philadelphia, Pa.: Lippincott Williams & Wilkins, 2006.

Berendt, Joachim-Ernst. *The World Is Sound: Nada Brahma*. Rochester, Vt.: Destiny Books, 1991.

Briggs, George Weston. *Gorakhnath and the Kanphata Yogis*. New Delhi, India: Munshiram Manoharial Publishers, 1938.

Carrera, Reverend Jaganath. *Inside the Yoga Sutras*. Buckingham, Va.: Integral Yoga Publications, 2006.

Chinmayananda, Swami. *Self-Unfoldment*. Piercy, Calif.: Chinmaya Publications, 1992.

Desikachar, T. K. V. *The Heart of Yoga: Developing a Personal Practice*. Rochester, Vt.: Inner Traditions, 1995.

———. *Health, Healing, and Beyond: Yoga and the Living Tradition of T. Krishnamacharya*. New York: Aperture Foundation, 1998.

Donahaye, Guy and Eddie Stern. *Guruji: A Portrait of Sri K. Pattabhi Jois Through the Eyes of His Students*. New York: Farrar, Straus and Giroux, 2010.

Feuerstein, Georg. *The Yoga Tradition*. 3rd ed. Prescott, Ariz.: Hohm Press, 1998.

Gheranda. *The Gheranda Samhita*. Translated by James Mallinson. Woodstock, N.Y.: YogaVidya.com, 2004.

Gorakshanatha. *Siddha-Siddantapaddhati*. Edited by Dr. M. L. Gharote and Dr. G. K. Pai. Puna, India: The Lonavla Institute, 2005.

Høeg, Peter. *The Quiet Girl*. New York: Farrar, Straus and Giroux, 2007.

Hölzel, Britta K., James Carmody, Mark Vangela, Christina Congletona, Sita M. Yerramsettia, Tim Gard, and Sara W. Lazar. "Mindfulness Practice Leads to Increases in Regional Brain Gray Matter Density." *Psychiatry Research: Neuroimaging* 191, no. 1 (2011): 36-43.

Johari, Harish. *Chakras: Energy Centers of Transformation*. Rochester, Vt.: Destiny Books, 2000.

Jois, Sri K. Pattbhi. *Yoga Mala*. Translated by Eddie Stern. New York: Patanjali Yoga Shala, 1999.

Iyengar, B. K. S. *Light on Yoga*. Rev. ed. New York: Schocken Books, 1979.

Khan, Hazrat Inayat. *The Mysticism of Sound and Music*. Boston: Shambhala, 1991.

Krishnamacharya, Sri T. *Yoga Makaranda: The Essence of Yoga*. Translated by T. K. V. Desikachar. Mysore, Karnataka: Madurai C.M.V. Press, 1934.

Lama, Dalai. *Advice on Dying: And Living a Better Life*. Translated by Jeffery Hopkins. New York: Atria Books, 2002.

Lehrer, Jonah. *Imagine: How Creativity Works*. New York: Houghton Mifflin Harcourt, 2012.

Michael, Edward Salim. *The Law of Attention: Nada Yoga and the Way of Inner Vigilance*. Rochester, Vt.: Inner Traditions, 2010.

Mohan, A. G. *Krishnamacharya: His Life and Teachings*. Boston: Shambhala, 2010.

Muktananda, Swami. *Play of Consciousness*. South Fallsburg, N.Y.: SYDA Foundation, 1978.

———. *Satsang with Baba: Vol. 1 & 5*. South Fallsburg, N.Y.: SYDA Foundation, 1978.

Panini. *The Shiva Samhita*. Translated by James Mallinson. Woodstock, N.Y.: YogaVidya.com, 2007.

Patanjali. *The Essential Yoga Sutras of Patanjali*. Translation and commentary by Geshe Michael Roach and Christie McNally. New York: Doubleday, 2005.

———. *The Yoga Philosophy of Patanjali*. Commentary by Vyasa. Translated by Swami Hariharananda Aranya. Boston: Shambhala, 2003.

———. *The Yoga-Sutra of Patanjali*. Translation and commentary by Georg Feuerstein. Rochester, Vt.: Inner Traditions, 1989.

———. *The Yoga Sutras of Patanjali*. Translation and commentary by Chip Hartranft. Boston: Shambhala, 2003.

———. *The Yoga Sutras of Patanjali.* Translation and commentary by Sri Swami Satchidananda. Buckingham, Va.: Integral Yoga Publications Inc., 2003.

———. *The Yoga Sutras.* Translation and commentary by Edwin D. Bryant. New York: North Point Press, 2009.

———. *Light on the Yoga Sutras of Patanjali.* Translation and commentary by B. K. S. Iyengar. New York: HarperCollins, 1993.

Ramachandran, V. S. and E. M. Hubbard. "Synaesthesia—A Window Into Perception, Thought and Language." *Journal of Consciousness Studies* 8, no. 12 (2001): 3–34.

———. "The Phenomenology of Synaesthesia." *Journal of Consciousness Studies* 10, no. 8 (2003): 49–57.

Rinpoche, Sogyal. *The Tibetan Book of Living and Dying.* New York: HarperCollins, 1994.

Sambhava, Padma. *Tibetan Book of the Dead.* Translation and commentary by Steven Hodge. New Alresford, U.K.: Godsfield Press, 1999.

———. *Tibetan Book of the Dead: Liberation Through Understanding in the Between.* Translation and commentary by Robert Thurman. New York: Bantam Books, 1994.

Sankara, Adi. *Shankara's Crest-Jewel of Discrimination.* Translation and commentary by Swami Prabhavananda and Christopher Isherwood. Hollywood, Calif.: Vedanta Press, 1947.

———. *Yoga Sutra Bhashya Vivarana of Sankara: Vol. 1 & 2.* Critical notes and translation by T. S. Rukmani. New Delhi, India: Munshiram Manoharlal Publishers, 2001.

———. *Yoga Taravali.* Translation and commentary by T. K. V. Desikachar and Kausthub Desikachar. Chennai, India: Krishnamacharya Yoga Mandiram, 2003.

Sarasvati, Shri Brahmananda. *Nada Yoga: The Science, Psychology and Philosophy of Anahata Nada Yoga.* Monroe, N.Y.: Baba Bhagavandas Publication Trust, 1999.

———. *Supersonic and Ultrasonic Music: The Inner Inner Nadam, Sound Energy and Sound Current.* Monroe, N.Y.: Baba Bhagavandas Publication Trust, 1995.

Sivananda, Swami. *Tantra Yoga, Nada Yoga and Kriya Yoga.* 6th ed. Uttaranchai, Himalayas, India: The Divine Life Society, 2004.

———. *Music as Yoga.* 2nd ed. Uttaranchai, Himalayas, India: The Divine Life Society, 2007.

Stern, Eddie, and Deirde Summerbells. *Sri K. Pattabhi Jois: A Tribute.* New York: Eddie Stern and Gwyneth Paltrow, 2002.

Svatmarama, Swami. *Hathapradipika.* Translated by and commentary by Swami Kuvalayanandaji and Swami Digambaraji Akers. Pune, Maharashra, India: K.S.M.Y.M., 1970.

———. *The Hatha Yoga Pradipika.* Translation and commentary by Jyotsna of Brahmananda. Adyar, Chennai, India: The Adyar Library and Research Center, 1972.

———. *The Hatha Yoga Pradipika.* Translation and commentary by Swami Multibodhananda. Mungar, Bihar, India: Bihar School of Yoga, 1985.

———. *The Hatha Yoga Pradipika.* Translated by Brian Dana Akers. Woodstock, N.Y.: YogaVidya.com, 2002.

———. *The Hatha Yoga Pradipika.* Translated by Pancham Sinh. New Delhi, India: Munshiram Manoharial Publishers, 2007.

Upnaisad-Brahma-Yogin, S'ri. *The Yoga-Upanisads.* Translation and commentary by T. R. S'rinivasa Ayyangar. Adyar, Madras, India: The Vasanta Press, 1938.

DISCOGRAPHY

Cohen, Leonard. *The Essential Leonard Cohen,* "Anthem." New York: Sony BMG, 2002.

Coltrane, John. *The Art of John Coltrane,* "Equinox." New York: Atlantic, 1959.

Davis, Miles. *Kind of Blue,* "So What." New York: Columbia Records, 1959.

Eno, Brian, and Robert Fripp. *Morning Star,* "Wind on Water." Beverly Hills, Calif.: DGM, 2008.

Gould, Glenn. *The Idea of North.* Toronto, Ontario: Canadian Broadcasting Corporation, 1992.

Kunzel, Erich, and Cincinnati Pops. *The Stokowski Sound: Transcriptions for Orchestra by Leopold Stokowski,* "The Sunken Cathedral." Cleveland, Ohio: Telarc Records, 1990.

Reich, Steve. *Music for 18 Musicians.* ECM, 2000.

VIDEOGRAPHY

Campbell, Joseph. *Sukhavati*. Directed by Maxine Harris. Silver Spring, Md.: Acorn Media, 2005.

Girard, Francios. *Thirty-two Short Films about Glenn Gloud*. Sony Pictures, 1993.

Rose, Charlie. *The Brain Series*. New York: The Simons Foundation, PBS, 2012.

Swyer, Alan. *Spiritual Revolution*. East Meets West Productions (II), 2008.

WEBOGRAPHY

Cullen, Lisa Takeuchi. "How to Get Smarter, One Breath at a Time." *Time Magazine*, Jan. 10, 2006. www.time.com/time/magazine/article/0,9171,1147167,00.html.

Gross, Jason. "Perfect Sound Forever." Online Magazine presents Jon Hassell, 1997. www.moredarkthanshark.org/eno_int_perso-jul97.html.

Lama, Dalai, and Arianna Huffington. "Arianna and the Dalai Lama discuss sleep." http://on.aol.com/video/arianna-and-the-dalai-lama-discuss-sleep-517365946.

Williams, Monier. *Monier Williams Sanskrit-English Dictionary*, 2008. www.sanskrit-lexicon.uni-koeln.de/monier/.

Ramachandran, V. S. "3 Clues to Understanding Your Brain," TED, 2007. www.ted.com/talks/vilayanur_ramachandran_on_your_mind.html.

Stern, Eddie. "The Practice." Sri K. Pattabhi Jois Ashtanga Yoga Institute. http://kpjayi.org/the-practice.

Index

Audio List

The following sound samples can be found on YouTube. The links provided below were active at the time of publication. Should these Web addresses no longer work, please search on the identification information also provided below.

Chapter 6, page 32
"Collection of Chöömej Styles" by Oleg Kuular
http://youtu.be/F8hyMW6pskc

Chapter 10, page 42
"Bottlenose Dolphins" by Atmoji Kubesa
http://youtu.be/nTXG105QrWI

Chapter 11, page 45
"I Am Sitting in a Room" by Alvin Lucier
http://youtu.be/TSR2LSuzP_M

Chapter 12, page 47
"The Idea of North" by Glenn Gould
http://youtu.be/W6Hrl7-nDVE

Chapter 14, page 52
"Yamantaka puja" by Gyuto monks
http://youtu.be/Tf22JS9IGFs

Chapter 20, page 70
"Equinox" by John Coltrane
http://youtu.be/5m2HN2y0yV8

"So What" by Miles Davis
http://youtu.be/SPivuC4fzQY

Chapter 20, page 71

"La Cathédrale engloutie" ("Sunken Cathedral") by Claude Debussy
http://youtu.be/c9UKua69NSI

"Wind on Water" by Brian Eno
http://youtu.be/9xBwINSmTOs

"Music for 18 Musicians" by Steve Reich
http://youtu.be/BuP-c0U5TTc

Chapter 29, page 98

Ocean ("Sound of the Ocean")
http://youtu.be/WAGLE1X_drc

Thunder ("Extreme Close Lightning in HD Compilation! Loud Thunder!")
http://youtu.be/Sp9bKDHRfsM

Waterfall ("The Forest Waterfall HD—The Calming Sound of Water")
http://youtu.be/FF2bhR7s3VY

Drums ("Kodo 'O-Daiko' HD Japanese Drummers")
http://youtu.be/C7HL5wYqAbU

Large Bell ("Balzan [Malta] Parish Church")
http://youtu.be/gtc_oKRY7kI

Flute ("RagaChitram TV Show, Hindustani Flute, Steve Gorn")
http://youtu.be/ke5SMAi6yyg

Chimes ("Woodstock Emperor Harp")
http://youtu.be.com/watch?v=hJ2_rVJnZZ0

Bees ("15 HD Minutes Bees Flying In and Out of a Hive with Stereo Sound")
http://youtu.be/0iMsnKrADt4

Crickets ("Sounds of Night Crickets")
http://youtube.com/watch?v=jzN3yJXlWrg

Overtone singing ("'Dharana' by Baird Hersey & Prana")
http://youtu.be/5CyjpV_8bCc